Praise for the *Intelligent Patient Guide* series

The *Intelligent Patient Guide to Breast Cancer* walks you
through each step of your diagnosis, treatment and prognosis…
with explanations that are easily understood.
It brought everything together, making it so clear.

— J. McIntosh, Patient

As a patient advocate and breast cancer survivor,
I lend and use my copy of the *Intelligent Patient Guide* often.
The book helps equip patients to better understand the need
to take charge in the design of their own survival.

— B. Cameron

It was so informative. I felt so secure knowing what
was going to happen with every step.

— D. Powell, Patient

A tremendous tool that I make available to all my patients.

— Dr. J. Caines, Halifax, Nova Scotia

I found the *Intelligent Patient Guide* an excellent tool
during my recent surgery and treatments. It gave me a sense
of being an active participant on the road to recovery.

— S. Moorhouse, RN, Patient

Thank you for writing the *Intelligent Patient Guide*
to Breast Cancer. It is straightforward and easy to understand.
Specific passages particular to my own situation were easily
found. It is a most convenient clarification for myself,
family, and friends.

— D. Clarke, Patient

D0377357

The *Intelligent Patient Guide...* was at my side
for the eight months I fought breast cancer. When I needed
[information], it never failed me.

— Former CEO, Canadian Cancer Society and
National Cancer Institute of Canada

This book's clear, concise descriptions and especially its
empathetic style made it my only "book" companion
along the road of my treatments. I became not only informed
but also reassured and calmed.

— H. Thompson, Patient

The Intelligent Patient Guide To

Breast Cancer

Other books in the *Intelligent Patient Guide*
series include:

The Intelligent Patient Guide to Prostate Cancer, 3rd edition
by S. Larry Goldenberg, MD, Ian M. Thompson, MD
ISBN 0-9696125-5-9

The Intelligent Patient Guide to Colorectal Cancer, 2nd edition
by Michael E. Pezim, MD, David Owen, MB
ISBN 0-9696125-7-5

The Intelligent Patient Guide to Osteoporosis, 1st edition
by Roger A.L. Sutton, DM, Robert G. Josse, MB
ISBN 978-0-9811599-0-4

While the authors have made every effort to ensure that the material contained herein is accurate at time of publication, new discoveries or changes in treatment practices may ultimately invalidate some of the information presented here.

Intelligent Patient Guide Ltd.
Suite 30, 3195 Granville Street
Vancouver, British Columbia V6H 3K2
Canada
email: info@ipguide.com
fax: 604-876-9334

Library and Archives Canada Cataloguing in Publication

The intelligent patient guide to breast cancer / Ivo Olivotto ... [et al.]—5th ed.

(Intelligent patient guide)
Includes index.
Previous eds. written by Ivo Olivotto, Karen Gelmon, Urve Kuusk.
ISBN 0-9811599-1-1
978-0-9811599-1-1

    1. Breast—Cancer—Popular works. I. Olivotto, Ivo, 1956-
II. Series: Intelligent patient guide

RC280.B8I57 2011   616.99'449   C2011-906345-X

Cover design by POP Creative, Vancouver
Graphic production by Melissa Petrucha, Port Moody
Printed in Canada

This book is dedicated to the thousands of women who have lived and are living with breast cancer and who, through their stories and their strength, have taught us so much.

Authors

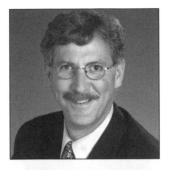

Ivo Olivotto, MD, FRCPC
Professor and
Head Division of Radiation Oncology
BC Cancer Agency and
University of British Columbia

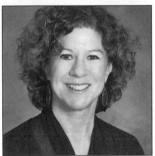

Karen Gelmon, MD, FRCPC
Professor
Division of Medical Oncology
BC Cancer Agency and
University of British Columbia

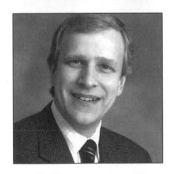

David McCready, MD, MSc, FRCSC, FACS
Professor of Surgery and
Gattuso Chair in Breast Surgical Oncology
Department of Surgical Oncology
University of Toronto

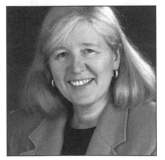

Urve Kuusk, MD, FRCPC
Clinical Associate Professor
Division of General Surgery
University of British Columbia

Contributing Authors

Judith Caldwell
Founder, Canadian Breast Cancer Foundation
British Columbia/Yukon Chapter

Paula Gordon, MD, FRCPC
Clinical Associate Professor
Department of Radiology
University of British Columbia

Susan Harris, PT, PhD
Professor Emerita
Department of Physical Therapy
University of British Columbia

Charmaine Kim-Sing, MD, FRCPC
Clinical Professor
Division of Radiation Oncology
BC Cancer Agency and University of British Columbia

Lis Smith, CCH
Clinical Hypnotherapist

Cheri Van Patten, MSc, RDN
Registered Dietician, Research Practitioner
BC Cancer Agency

Editor
Jay Draper

Illustrator
Jane Rowlands

Coordinator
Nicola Sutton, MBA

Series Medical Director
Michael E. Pezim, MD, FRCSC

Why read this book?

AFTER YOU HEAR THE WORDS "you have breast cancer" you may be in a state of shock. Despite this, you will be expected to make a series of major decisions, often in a hurry. "Should I have a mastectomy? Should I have reconstruction? Should I have radiation? Chemotherapy? Hormone therapy?" The choices seem so complicated. Women often end up wondering, "Should I just leave the decisions up to my doctors and do whatever they suggest?"

We believe not. Time and again we have seen that the patient who takes an active part in making the decisions that affect the course of her treatment is better able to cope than the patient who delegates control to her doctors. While we are not advocating that you make choices independent of your care providers' recommendations, we encourage you to become one of the decision-makers.

Since first publishing this book in 1995 and updating it in 1998, 2001, and 2006, we have been gratified to hear from many patients who have found the information useful. It has helped them understand the disease, ask doctors the questions that need to be asked, and make the decisions they need to make about their treatment.

Progress is continuous. Sometimes progress is sudden and dramatic but more often it is slow and incremental. As a result, as soon as a book is written there may be aspects of care that change or come into question. As much as we regret these discrepancies, we applaud any progress that will improve care for women with breast cancer.

It is important to note that the statistics we have quoted about risks and prognosis refer to the general or "average" situation. Special additional circumstances may modify your individual risk and need to be discussed with your doctor. And remember, everyone's story is a bit different.

We hope this book can help you move through the fear, to a place of hope and strength and the promise of life ahead—in spite of breast cancer.

Ivo Olivotto, MD
Karen Gelmon, MD
David McCready, MD
Urve Kuusk, MD

Table of Contents

Why read this book? xi

PART 1   *Breast cancer:*
What is it? How is it detected? 1

SECTION 1   **What is breast cancer?** 3
     1. What is cancer? 5
     2. How common is breast cancer? 9
     3. What causes breast cancer? 12
     4. Prevention—Is it possible? 20

SECTION 2   **The normal breast** 25
     5. Breast anatomy and function 27

SECTION 3   **Methods to detect breast cancer** 33
     6. Options for breast screening 35

SECTION 4   **What do I do when I find a lump?** 43
     7. A visit to the doctor 45
     8. Breast lumps and other problems 47
     9. Diagnostic mammograms, ultrasounds,
        MRI scans, and PET scans 50
     10. Biopsies 58
     11. If the screening mammogram is abnormal 65

SECTION 5   **What type of cancer is it?** 69
     12. The pathology report:
        Reading the cancer's telltale signs 71
     13. In situ cancer:
        Cancer that has not invaded or spread 76
     14. The different types
        of invasive breast cancer 80

PART 2   *What are my options now that*
            I have a diagnosis of breast cancer? 87

SECTION 6   **An overview of treatment** 89
            15. An overview of breast cancer treatment 91
            16. Staging and prognosis 93
            17. Strategies for navigating the
                cancer care system 98

SECTION 7   **The surgical options** 103
            18. The doctor has suggested surgery:
                What should I do? 105
            19. Types of breast surgery 107
            20. What type of surgery is best for me? 116
            21. Hospitalization and recovering
                from surgery 121

SECTION 8   **Preventing recurrence of cancer** 127
            22. Additional treatment following surgery:
                Radiation, chemotherapy, and
                hormone treatment 129
            23. Treatment of in situ breast cancer 132

SECTION 9   **Radiation therapy** 139
            24. Radiation therapy: What is it? 141
            25. Who benefits from radiation therapy? 147
            26. Side effects of radiation therapy 152

SECTION 10 **Hormone therapy** 157
            27. Hormone therapy:
                What is it and who benefits from it? 159
            28. Side effects of hormone therapy 165

SECTION 11 **Chemotherapy** 173
            29. Chemotherapy: What is it? 175
            30. Who benefits from chemotherapy? 180
            31. Side effects of chemotherapy 185

PART 3   *Beyond the initial phase of treatment* 199

SECTION 12 **Coping with cancer** 201
            32. Living with a diagnosis of breast cancer:
                Tips for you, your family, and your friends ... 203
            33. Exercise, physical therapy,
                and management of lymphedema 214
            34. Reconstructive surgery 225

SECTION 13 **Lifestyle issues** 235
            35. Nutrition 237
            36. Stress and relaxation 249

SECTION 14 **What if cancer recurs?** 253
            37. Follow-up: Support, side effects,
                and concerns about recurrence 255
            38. Treatment of a local or regional recurrence ... 261
            39. Treatment of recurrence
                elsewhere in the body (metastasis) 264

SECTION 15 **Special topics** 273
            40. Breast cancer and pregnancy 275
            41. Breast cancer in young women 279
            42. Inherited breast cancer and genetic testing 282
            43. Male breast cancer 287
            44. Complementary and alternative treatments ... 288
            45. Clinical research:
                Looking for better answers 296
            46. Awareness and advocacy 299

APPENDIX   **Breast self-examination technique** 306

GLOSSARY 308

ADDITIONAL READING 316

INDEX 322

PART ONE | **Breast cancer:
What is it?
How is it detected?**

What is breast cancer?

CHAPTER ONE

What is cancer?

TO UNDERSTAND CANCER, it is important to learn about normal growth in the body.

How does the body grow and maintain itself?

The body is made up of billions of tiny cells. During normal growth, a cell becomes larger, and then divides into two "daughter" cells (Figure 1). After a period of time, each of these cells divides again. Our bodies experience a lot of wear and tear so old or worn out cells constantly need to be replaced. Normally this happens in an orderly way because each cell carries genetic instructions that regulate how fast the cell should divide and grow and when the cell should die. A balance between cells growing and dying keeps our bodies functioning normally.

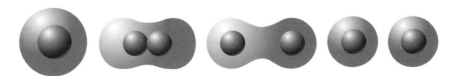

Figure 1: Normal cell division. A cell grows a bit larger and then divides into two cells.

When cell growth goes out of control

Benign growths

Sometimes cells disregard the normal balance between cell growth and death. As a result, a small, harmless lump of cells called a *benign* growth may form. A benign growth can occur in any part of the body.

Malignant growths

In other cases, cells may grow into a large mass or spread to other areas of the body. Cells that have this aggressive behaviour are called *malignant*. More commonly, a mass of such cells is called a *cancer* or a *carcinoma*. Cancer cells have some unique characteristics including the ability to travel in the blood stream. When clumps of cancer cells spread to other parts of the body, they are called *metastases*. Eventually, if a cancer grows unchecked it can overwhelm and destroy the part of the body or organ where it is located.

Cancer cells also have the ability to stimulate the development of blood vessels to increase their own blood supply and enhance their growth. This is called *angiogenesis*. Sometimes, a cancer may outgrow its oxygen and nutrient supply, and when this happens, a part of the cancer may suddenly die. The death of a group of cells within a cancer is known as *necrosis*.

Cancer cells have the ability to spread

Normal cells remain in the area of the body where they belong and do not spread to other parts of the body. However, cancer cells can invade into the blood vessels and spread (metastasize) to other parts of the body. The paths of spread include direct invasion and destruction of the organ of origin, spread through the lymphatic system, and spread through the blood stream to distant organs such as the lungs, liver, brain, or bones (Figure 2).

The original cancer in the breast is called the *primary* cancer. A cancer that has spread to another site is called a *secondary* or *metastatic* cancer.

When a cancer spreads, it retains most of the properties of the original cancer. This means that a breast cancer that has spread to the bones is still a breast cancer. Under the microscope it still looks like breast cancer and looks different than a cancer that started in the bone. When a breast cancer has spread it continues to behave like a breast cancer, not a cancer from the organ to which it has spread, for instance the lung or bone. When breast cancer cells spread, it is possible that some changes may occur in their genetic makeup and therefore sometimes metastases are biopsied to see if they still look identical to the primary.

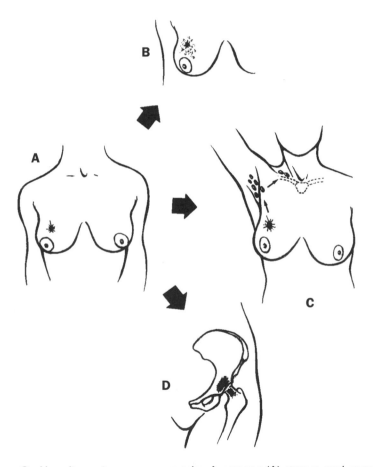

Figure 2: How breast cancer spreads. A cancer (A) grows and spreads by direct local invasion (B) of the breast itself or (C) through the lymphatic system to lymph nodes or (D) through the blood stream to distant organs such as the bones, lungs, liver, or brain.

Breast cancer does not develop overnight

It can take years of cells dividing before a normal cell becomes recognized as a cancer cell. The progression from normal cell to cancer cell is due to the accumulation of small genetic changes in the cell. Under the microscope these genetic changes are reflected in changes in the appearance of the cell. At first there are very small changes that may not be detectable, then cells may appear slightly abnormal or *atypical*. The cell may also begin to divide, grow more quickly and accumulate in excessive numbers (hyperplasia). Then, over the years, these cells continue to change, appear more abnormal looking and finally become recognized as cancerous (Figure 3).

Initially the cancer cells are confined within the milk ducts of the breast (*in situ* cancer), but with time, the cells develop the ability to invade through the milk duct wall (an *invasive* cancer) and eventually into the blood vessels or lymphatic system.

Present technology cannot detect one or even a few cancer cells. It is only possible to detect small lumps of cancer cells. By the time a cancer is detected as a 1 cm lump, it contains about one billion cells and has likely been growing for 2 to 8 years.

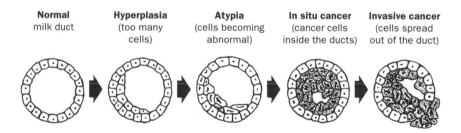

Normal milk duct	**Hyperplasia** (too many cells)	**Atypia** (cells becoming abnormal)	**In situ cancer** (cancer cells inside the ducts)	**Invasive cancer** (cells spread out of the duct)

Figure 3: Breast cancer does not develop overnight. Cells gradually become more abnormal-looking or *atypical* (see text). Eventually, the cells are recognized as being sufficiently abnormal to be called cancer cells. They are initially inside the milk ducts (*in situ* cancer) and later develop into invasive breast cancer.

CHAPTER TWO

How common is breast cancer?

BREAST CANCER IS THE MOST COMMON TYPE of cancer in women. Each year approximately 23,500 new cases of breast cancer are diagnosed in Canada (200 in men) and there are over 5,000 deaths from breast cancer. There are approximately ten times that number of new cases and deaths from breast cancer each year in the US. Breast cancer accounts for 4% of all deaths among women in North America each year and the loss of thousands of productive years of life.

"One in nine" is misleading

One often hears that "one in nine" women will get breast cancer. The trouble with this figure is that it can be misleading because the risk of breast cancer increases with age. A woman at age 70, for example, is four times more likely to get breast cancer in a given year than a woman who is 40 years old. The ratio "one in nine" refers to the chance that a woman will develop breast cancer if she lives to the age of 90. Since many women die of other causes before the age of 90, they don't actually reach the age group at highest risk.

Recent changes in the incidence of breast cancer

The number of new cases diagnosed each year per 100,000 women is called the *incidence*. From the 1940s to very recently, there has been a slow but steady increase in the number of new cases of breast cancer diagnosed each year in North America. This increase has been attributed to changes in nutrition, such as consumption of more calories, the use of hormone replacement therapy, and changes in reproductive patterns. Today, women start menstruating several years earlier, delay having babies and have fewer children than they did in a century ago. These factors tend to increase exposure of the maturing breast to estrogens and have been linked to the higher rates of breast cancer.

In addition, there was a definite increase in the incidence of breast cancer (more than 1% per year) reported in the mid-1980s. That was largely due to the increased use of screening mammograms, which can detect some cancers 2 to 5 years before a lump can be felt by the woman or her doctor. As most women had at least one mammogram during the 1980s and 1990s, the sudden wave of earlier detected cancers passed, and the incidence rates dropped back to the background rate prior to the screening era.

In the last few years there has been a suggestion of a decreased incidence in the number of cases of breast cancer that has been attributed to the decreasing use of hormone replacement therapy after menopause.

You can estimate your own risk

Rather than considering a lifetime risk to age 90, a more useful question is: "What is my risk, given my current age?"

Table 1 shows the average risk each year of developing breast cancer for typical North American women at specific ages. Using Table 1, based on her current age, the "average" woman can estimate her risk of developing breast cancer over the next year. The risk over the next decade is 10 times the annual risk. For example, if you are 42, your annual risk is slightly higher than that of the 40-year-old listed in Table 1, say 1/1,000 per year. Over the next decade your risk would be 10 x 1/1,000 = 1/100 or approximately 1% over the next 10 years. This risk is much easier to live with than one in nine.

Table 1	Annual risk of developing breast cancer
At age	**Risk**
30 years	1 in 6,000 per year
40 years	1 in 1,200 per year
50 years	1 in 550 per year
60 years	1 in 400 per year
70 years	1 in 300 per year
80 years	1 in 250 per year

Table 2 shows not the annual risk, but the lifetime risk up to certain ages. As you can see from Table 2, even a woman who is 75 years old does not yet have a "one in nine" chance of developing breast cancer. More specific, individualized risk estimates can be determined by considering additional factors that are associated with a higher risk of developing breast cancer, and then multiplying the "average" risk at a certain age by the risk factor. A web-based model to calculate the 5-year and lifetime risk of developing breast cancer for an individual woman can be found at: www.cancer.gov/bcrisktool/. Chapter 3 discusses some of the causes of breast cancer and ranks them according to their importance.

Table 2	Chance of developing breast cancer by a given age
Age	**Risk to this age**
by 25 years	less than 1 in 1,000
by 50 years	1 in 63
by 75 years	1 in 15
by 90 years	1 in 9

CHAPTER THREE

What causes breast cancer?

Why me?

"WHY DID I GET BREAST CANCER?" This is a question that doctors can almost never answer with any certainty. However, it is not your "fault" or "punishment" for something you did or did not do, and it is not something you subconsciously "needed."

There has been a lot of controversy over the years about the possible causes of breast cancer: diet, hormones, genetic make-up, or substances in the environment. Today we realize that there is no single factor that causes breast cancer, but that it is a combination of things, some more important than others. The relative importance of genetics, lifestyle, and the environment varies between individual women.

What is a risk factor?

A *risk factor* refers to something that increases your chance of getting a disease, in this case, breast cancer. A strong risk factor greatly increases the chance, while a weak risk factor just slightly increases your chance. For example, in the case of lung cancer, smoking is a very strong risk factor since a smoker is far more likely to get lung cancer than a non-smoker.

With breast cancer there are several known risk factors, ranging from strong to weak (see Table 3).

A *strong* risk factor is defined as something that increases the chance of developing breast cancer by more than four times compared to someone without this risk factor. *Moderate* means an increase of two to four times the risk, and *weak* means less than two times the risk.

Table 3	**Risk factors associated with the development of breast cancer**	
Strong (Risk is 4 times higher for those with compared to without the factor)	**Moderate** (Risk 2 to 4 times higher for those with compared to without the factor)	**Weak** (Risk 1 to 2 times higher for those with compared to without the factor)
Female sex	Over 30 years old at birth of first child	Oral contraceptive use
Advancing age (age 70 or greater compared to age 40 or younger)	Past breast biopsy showing atypical cells or hyperplasia	First menstrual period before the age of 12 years
Previous breast cancer (especially lobular carcinoma)	Postmenopausal obesity	Menopause after the age of 54 years
Family history of breast or ovarian cancer, particularly if premenopausal, in both breasts or numerous family members		Family history of breast cancer if the affected relatives were all older or postmenopausal
Increased breast density as defined on a mammogram or MRI		Prolonged postmenopausal hormone use
Past breast biopsy showing severely abnormal cells and hyperplasia		Diet, obesity
		Moderate to heavy alcohol consumption
		Repeated chest X-rays in younger women

Strong risk factors

Increasing age is a strong risk factor for developing breast cancer. Women who are 50 years old have double the risk of women who are 40, and the risk doubles again by the age of 70 years (see Table 1, page 11). For three-quarters of the women who get breast cancer, being female and getting older are the only identifiable risk factors. The remaining 25% of women with breast cancer have a combination of other risk factors.

Previous history of breast cancer

Most women who get one breast cancer do not get another. However, every year about one in every 200 women with a first breast cancer will develop a new cancer in the opposite breast. Women with the lobular type of breast cancer (Chapter 14) have a higher chance, about 1% per year, of getting cancer in the opposite breast. Taking an anticancer hormone drug like tamoxifen or an aromatase inhibitor (Arimidex, Femara, or Aromasin—see Chapter 27) reduces the chance of developing a second cancer. However, it is still important to keep the second breast under surveillance with regular self and physician examinations and a yearly mammogram (breast X-ray).

Family history of breast cancer

A family history of breast cancer in a close relative such as your mother, sister, or daughter contributes to your risk. However, breast cancer in only one distant relative such as an aunt or grandmother may have little or no impact on your risk. A history of breast cancer in a premenopausal close relative, breast cancer or ovarian cancer (or both) in more than one close relative, or cancer in both breasts of a close relative confers a four to six times higher risk of developing breast cancer compared to a woman of the same age who does not have relatives with breast cancer.

In some families an increased risk of developing breast cancer may be passed on by a specific genetic mutation. For example, families with an inherited mutation in the BRCA1 or BRCA2 gene have a tendency to develop both breast and ovarian cancer. Women who inherit such a mutation have a lifetime risk of developing breast cancer as high as 85%. Many of these families are characterized by breast cancer developing before the age of 50, both breast and ovary cancer in family members, or breast cancer occurring in male relatives. These mutations can be inherited through either your mother or father and may occur in any ethnic group (see Chapter 42).

Increased breast density

Breasts are composed of glandular (milk glands and ducts) and fatty tissue (see Chapter 5). The amount of glandular tissue is high in young women and women who are pregnant or lactating. As women age, the glandular breast tissue is gradually replaced by fat. Women who have a very high proportion of their breast tissue composed of dense glands are at higher risk of developing a breast cancer. This may be related to hormonal or genetic factors that cause a greater stimulation of the breast glands and predispose the breast cells to form cancers. It is also more difficult to detect a small cancer in a very dense breast compared to a fatty one. As a result, if the breasts are very dense on a mammogram, other tests such as an ultrasound or magnetic resonance image (MRI) may be necessary (see Chapter 6).

Moderate risk factors

Later pregnancy

The delivery of a first child before the age of 20 causes hormonal changes in the breast tissue that provide modest protection against breast cancer. Delaying the first child until after the age of 30 or having no full-term pregnancies increases a woman's risk of developing breast cancer by two to four times. Breastfeeding decreases the chance of getting breast cancer by a small amount. In cultures where women breast feed each child for three or four years, this effect may be much greater.

Previous breast biopsy showing abnormal cells or excessive accumulation of cells

As described in Chapter 1, a normal cell becomes a cancer cell through a series of changes in which the cells begin to divide and accumulate in excessive numbers (*hyperplasia*), become abnormal (*atypia*) and finally develop into cancer cells. If hyperplasia is seen in tissue removed during a breast biopsy, especially when there is both atypia and hyperplasia, the woman has a two to four times greater chance of developing breast cancer compared to a woman without these changes. If there is severe atypia and hyperplasia, especially in a woman who also has a family history of breast cancer, an eight-fold increased risk can be expected.

Weak risk factors

There have been conflicting results about oral contraceptives but it appears that using these medications for more than 10 years does confer a weak increased risk of breast cancer. In contrast, oral contraceptive use *decreases* the risk of ovarian cancer. Modern oral contraceptives have a lower estrogen content, and should have an even smaller impact on the risk of developing breast cancer. Overall the risk from modern oral contraceptives is very minimal and their use needs to be balanced in the light of other health benefits.

The onset of menstrual periods before the age of 12 years and cessation of menstruation after the age of 54 years weakly increase the risk of breast cancer.

Postmenopausal estrogen

The risk associated with postmenopausal hormone use (hormone replacement therapy) is controversial. Overall, women who have at some point used postmenopausal estrogens, alone or in combination with progesterone, have a modestly higher chance of developing breast cancer as compared with women who have never used these medications. Women who have taken postmenopausal hormones for longer than seven to 10 years have an approximately 1.5-fold increased risk compared to non-users. This modestly higher breast cancer risk has to be considered in context with the potentially beneficial effects of these medications, including, among other things, a lower risk of bone fractures and relief of hot flushes, vaginal dryness, and mood swings that may accompany menopause. In large studies the combination of estrogen and progesterone caused a greater increased risk than estrogen alone. There is insufficient data to comment on the risk from products with progesterone alone. Bio-identical hormones are considered to have the same effects on breast cancer risk as synthetic hormones because even the hormones produced naturally in the body are associated with an increased risk of developing breast cancer.

Diet, body weight, body mass index, hip/waist ratio, and exercise

There has been extensive research into the role of diet in the formation of breast cancer. Some authorities believe that up to 30% of breast cancers may be attributable to dietary influences.

Studies of populations that move from an area of low breast cancer risk (e.g., Japan) to an area of high risk (e.g., North America) show that within one to two generations the migrant population adopts the risk level of the new country. This is thought to be due to changes of diet and lifestyle that the children and grandchildren of the immigrants adopt.

It is not clear which specific dietary factors are important in causing breast cancer but the principal culprit has been thought to be overall dietary calories and fat. Furthermore, it is not known which type of dietary fat may be the culprit: saturated or unsaturated, fat of vegetable or animal origin, or whether the effect is simply related to eating too many calories.

Obesity and an increase in body mass index (BMI) are associated with an increased breast cancer risk in the postmenopausal years. This may relate to the hormonal changes that occur in the body with obesity including changes in how the body responds to insulin. The impact of body weight on the risk of developing breast cancer however is complicated. Women who are markedly underweight in the premenopausal years also experience an increased risk of breast cancer.

Studies have suggested that the shape of one's body also contributes. Women with a high waist-to-hip ratio, that is, carrying one's weight and fat in one's middle, have a greater risk for breast cancer compared to women with other body shapes.

Moderate to heavy alcohol consumption (more than three drinks or six glasses of wine or beer per week) has been associated with a weak increase in the risk of developing breast cancer. It remains reasonable to have an occasional drink or glass of wine, but there are studies that suggest that even minimal alcohol carries a risk. This must be put in the context of other health conditions that may benefit from minimal alcohol.

Studies of exercise have also been contradictory but in general it is thought to be of benefit. Most of this benefit may relate to BMI and body fat composition.

Environmental factors

Radiation from X-rays is a common concern. Even at low doses, the use of repeated chest X-rays in younger women (younger than age 20 years) has been associated with an increased risk of breast cancer. The usual dose of radiation from a mammogram (X-ray of the breast) is very small. Since routine mammograms tend to be used in women older than 40 years and since older individuals tend to be more resistant to the effects of radiation, the chance that a mammogram will cause a breast cancer is very low. Most authorities estimate that the small risk of causing a breast cancer is considerably less than the benefit that a mammogram may offer by revealing breast cancer earlier (see Chapter 6). Women who have had significant radiation exposure at an early age due to other health problems have a higher risk of developing breast cancer. Such women include those who had curative radiation therapy as treatment for Hodgkin's lymphoma or thyroid cancer, and women who had repeated X-rays for spinal or chest problems.

Chemical carcinogens are everywhere in our environment, but no specific chemical or substance has been identified as specifically causing a greater number of breast cancers. Although there has been concern about organochlorines found in pesticides, so far no direct association has been proven between the use of pesticides and the incidence of breast cancer.

Studies of the effect of smoking on the risk of developing breast cancer have been controversial. However, there is a weak association between exposure to both primary and secondary smoke and the risk of developing breast cancer. Younger women and girls with developing breasts may be at a greater risk from exposure to cigarette smoke than older women.

Race: Little if any effect on risk

Historically, in the US, black women have had a lower incidence of breast cancer than white women, but unfortunately the survival rate for black women is lower than the survival rate for white women. This has been attributed to differences in access to medical care or differences in the type of breast cancer that develop in black women. In Canada, the age-adjusted risk among First Nations women seems to be lower than among Caucasian women.

Ethnic groups who migrate to North America from areas of low risk (e.g., Japan and Southeast Asia) adopt the higher risk of the "average" woman in North America within one to two generations. This strongly suggests that the influences of race and ethnic background have little if any role compared to diet, lifestyle, or other environmental factors.

Chapter Four

Prevention—Is it possible?

Risk factors we cannot change

IT IS FRUSTRATING that the major known risk factors for developing breast cancer cannot be changed, such as female sex, advancing age, family or previous personal history of breast cancer, and the age at which menstrual periods begin (see Chapter 3). Getting pregnant at a very young age may have a weak protective effect but there are many reasons why delaying pregnancy may be more important.

Risk and health factors that we can change

Lifestyle factors

Lifestyle changes have been shown to reduce the chance of developing heart attacks, strokes, and some cancers. Some studies indicate that regular exercise (4 hours or more per week) or heavy manual labor at work can reduce the chance of getting breast cancer. It is not known why this happens, whether it is due to changes in hormone levels which occur with vigorous exercise, athletes' eating habits, or perhaps the different amounts of body fat carried by active and inactive women. This area requires further study, but several hours per week of regular exercise is encouraged.

Stress has many different meanings and personal interpretations but usually involves a sense of loss of control or low self-esteem.

Making positive changes to reduce your personal level of stress can have substantial health benefits but may not affect cancer risk.

Diet

Diet is clearly an important factor in the development of breast cancer and is something you can change. However, there is no specific diet that can guarantee that breast cancer will not develop. There is no simple remedy to prevent breast cancer in spite of what one reads on the newsstands. A healthy diet consists of reducing your total amount of calories taken and reducing the proportion of calories taken as fat to between 20 and 30% of your total calorie intake. This can be achieved by trimming the visible fat from meat, using leaner cuts, limiting pastries and chocolate, avoiding sauces rich in fat or cream, and substituting low-fat milk products (skim or 1%) for the higher fat alternatives. In a large Canadian study, women who intentionally severely restricted their fat intake did not have any lower risk of breast cancer than women who followed their usual diet. Increasing the amount of green and yellow vegetables, which contain vitamin A, and the fibre content of the diet, is encouraged (see Chapter 35). A balanced diet without excess calories or processed foods is recommended. Drinking less alcohol may be beneficial. Women who consume more than three drinks or six glasses of beer or wine per week have an increased chance of developing breast cancer.

Hormones

Moderate use of oral contraceptives and postmenopausal estrogens may have more advantages with respect to general health than disadvantages in terms of breast cancer risk. Limiting postmenopausal estrogen use to less than 10 years will reduce the chance of getting breast cancer.

Tamoxifen, an anti-estrogen drug, is used for some types of breast cancer (see Chapter 27). A large North American study tested the value of tamoxifen as a method of preventing breast cancer. Over 13,000 women who had five times higher than the normal risk of developing breast cancer volunteered for this study. Half the women took tamoxifen daily for 5 years and the other half took an inactive placebo tablet daily. Tamoxifen was shown to reduce the chance of developing breast cancer by about 40% and also reduce the risk of hip fractures, but increased the chance of developing blood clots in the legs and lungs and the chance of getting cancer of the endometrium (uterus). The aromotase inhibitor exemestane (Aromasin, see Chapter 27), has similarly been shown to reduce the risk of developing breast cancer by 40 to 50%, but increases the risk of osteoporosis and fractures. Tamoxifen or exemestane are not recommended as prevention for all women. However, for a woman at very high risk of developing breast cancer (those at more than five times the average risk), taking an anti-estrogen for five years may have more benefits than risks. Women should discuss their individual risk of breast cancer and the likelihood of complications from tamoxifen or an aromotase inhibitor with their doctors. A breast cancer risk assessment tool can be found at www.cancer.gov/bcrisktool.

Raloxifene, an anti-estrogen drug used for osteoporosis, has also been studied as a breast cancer prevention agent. Raloxifene reduced the chance of developing breast cancer and had a lower risk of developing endometrial cancer compared to tamoxifen, but both caused hot flushes and other menopausal side effects. Aromatase inhibitors such as Arimidex (anastrosole) and Aromasin (exemestane) are also being studied as prevention drugs for post-menopausal women.

Surgical prevention

Rarely, a family may have numerous cases of breast cancer including several members of each generation affected. Much research is now aimed at identifying specific genes that will indicate which women in these families have an extremely high risk of developing breast cancer. Two such genes, called *BRCA1* and *BRCA2*, were discovered in 1994. Women who have inherited mutations in the BRCA1 gene have a 50 to 85% lifetime chance of developing breast cancer and a 45% lifetime chance of developing ovarian cancer. Women with BRCA2 mutations have a high risk of breast cancer, as do men in the family, but a lower, yet still significant, risk of ovarian cancer. (Chapter 42 discusses family risks and genetic testing in more detail.)

Surgical prevention (removal of both breasts) may be considered by women with a very high risk (lifetime risk of 50% or higher) of developing breast cancer who have participated in counselling and weighed the alternatives carefully. This procedure is called *prophylactic mastectomy*. If both breasts are to be removed as a preventive measure all the underlying breast tissue should be removed. It is not necessary to remove the lymph nodes. Mastectomy substantially reduces the chance of developing a later breast cancer but a small risk remains because 100% of the breast glandular tissue cannot be removed. Some glandular tissue may remain against the skin or muscles of the chest wall.

If a mastectomy is chosen, it may be an advantage to do an immediate reconstruction (see Chapter 34). Subcutaneous mastectomy is a procedure in which the breast tissue is cut out through a small incision under each breast but the nipple and skin of the breast are not removed. Studies have shown that this procedure may leave behind 10 to 15% of the breast glandular tissue, so the risk of breast cancer is not eliminated. If the decision is taken to use a surgical approach to breast cancer prevention, eliminating as much of the breast tissue as possible is the goal, so total mastectomy with or without reconstruction is recommended.

The normal breast

CHAPTER FIVE

Breast anatomy and function

MOST PEOPLE DON'T REALIZE how extensive the breast is. Breast tissue can be found as high as the collarbone (clavicle) and extends from almost the middle of the chest over the breastbone (sternum) to the armpit (axilla) (Figure 4).

What is in the breast?

The breast consists of milk glands, fat, fibrous tissue, blood vessels, nerves and tubes (ducts) that, during lactation, carry milk from the breast glands to the nipple.

Breast milk is produced in hundreds of thousands of tiny glands (lobules) within the breast (Figure 5). These are drained by small ducts. The clusters of milk glands look like tiny bunches of grapes. From each lobule, larger ducts carry the milk to the nipple. The nipple surface contains about 20 duct openings, each draining a different part of the breast. All the milk glands are cushioned by fat. The normal lumps that can be felt in your breast are a combination of the milk glands, fat, and other fibrous tissues.

The proportion of milk glands, ducts, and fat in the breast changes as a woman grows older. During puberty, and as the breast develops, it consists mainly of ducts. In a 20-year-old woman, most of the breast is made up of milk glands. During pregnancy and breastfeeding (lactation), the glandular content of the breast

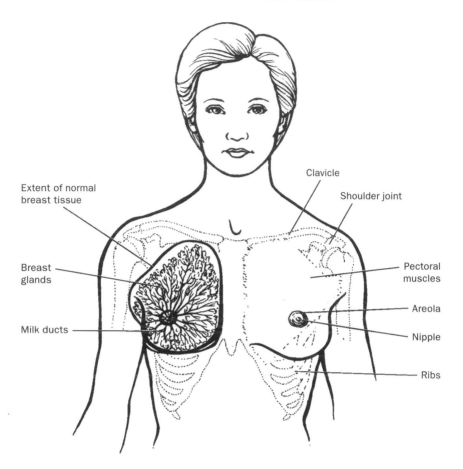

Figure 4: Extent of normal breast tissue and important underlying structures.

increases dramatically as the breast prepares to produce milk.

The fat content increases as you age, especially after menopause. In an elderly woman, almost all the breast is fatty tissue. Hormones taken after menopause tend to maintain the glandular tissue and delay the normal replacement of the breast glandular tissue by fat.

Ligaments help hold the breast in place

Throughout the breast there are many supporting ligaments, which are like thin but strong elastic bands. These ligaments are

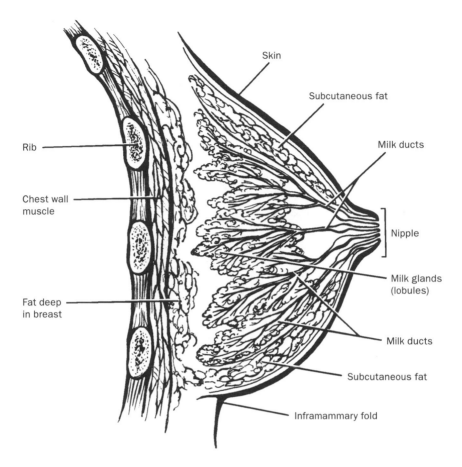

Skin

Subcutaneous fat

Milk ducts

Rib

Chest wall
muscle

Nipple

Fat deep
in breast

Milk glands
(lobules)

Milk ducts

Subcutaneous fat

Inframammary fold

Figure 5: A cross-sectional view of the breast showing the internal appearance of the breast and its relationship to the chest wall.

attached to the breast bone or muscles under the breast. With age, the ligaments tend to stretch and the normal breast begins to sag.

Muscles around the breast

A large, fan-shaped muscle lies beneath most of the breast. This is the pectoralis major muscle, which is responsible for some of the shoulder and arm movements. If you tense your arm and push in with your hand on your hip, you can feel this muscle as a firm ridge extending from the outside edge of the breast toward the armpit.

The pectoralis minor muscle is smaller and not readily felt because it is underneath the pectoralis major muscle.

Lymph nodes: where infection fighting occurs

The purpose of the lymphatic system is to fight infections in the body. There are tiny lymph vessels in every organ and tissue of the body. Fluid, which normally leaks from blood vessels to bathe body tissues, is collected by the lymph vessels and carried to groups of lymph nodes located in various places throughout the body. In the lymph nodes, infections and dead cells are "filtered out" and destroyed, and the "treated" fluid then enters the blood stream.

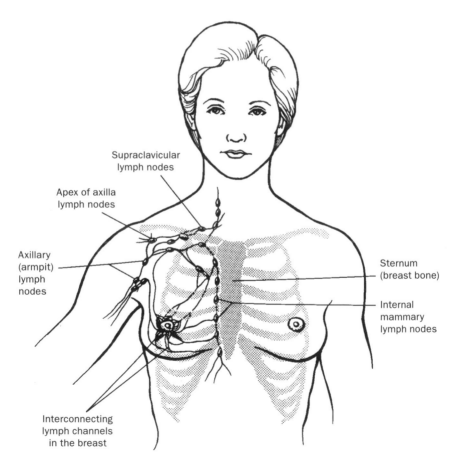

Figure 6: System of lymph nodes that drain the breast.

Figure 6 shows the location of the main groups of lymph nodes that drain the breast. They are just above the armpit, above and below the collarbone, and along the sternum (the internal mammary lymph nodes). There are between 30 and 50 lymph nodes in each armpit.

Lymph nodes are of particular importance in breast cancer because cancer cells sometimes enter the lymphatic vessels that drain the breast and can be carried to the lymph nodes where they settle and grow. Although we now realize that the type of breast cancer affects the risk of recurrence, it is still important to determine if any cancer cells are found in the lymph nodes at the time of diagnosis as this may affect the type of treatment that is recommended (see Chapter 14).

Sensation and the nerves around the breast

Many nerves pass through the breast to the skin and to the nipple. In addition, the intercostal-brachial nerves extend from the area between the ribs, through the armpit (axilla) to the underside or back of the upper arm. These nerves may be stretched or cut during surgery in the armpit, which leads to an unpleasant tingling, burning, numb or "thick" sensation on the back or underside of the upper arm. These sensations usually fade partly or completely over several months after surgery, but some numbness is often permanent.

Methods to detect breast cancer

Chapter Six

Options for breast screening

Screening is the use of a test to detect disease in an otherwise healthy individual. The goal of screening for breast cancer is to reduce the number of women dying from breast cancer by finding early cancers that are so small that they have not had a chance to spread beyond the breast. These breast cancers are usually too small to feel and are often cured by effective therapy directed to the breast (surgery or surgery plus radiation therapy).

Are screening mammograms useful?

For a screening test to be useful, it should be low-cost, relatively painless, widely available, safe, and relatively good at finding the disease. The disease that is being looked for should be common enough in the general population and be sufficiently life-threatening to justify doing the test on all the people being screened. In addition, there should be effective treatment available for the disease if it is found. Mammograms to detect early breast cancer meet all the criteria to be useful as a breast cancer-screening test.

A lot of research has examined different screening tests including mammograms, ultrasound, MRI, and breast self-examination. The recommendations of which tests to do, for whom, starting when, and how often, are revised as information becomes available over time. It is understandably confusing that different organizations have different recommendations as to what age women should start screening mammography, and how often they should be screened. Some of these differences are because different studies were used to decide policy or because the study data were interpreted differently. Some organizations base their recommendations on older studies with longer follow-up, while others consider more recent studies. The following is an explanation of the history of the studies of breast screening. If it's more detail than you want, skim or skip to the next section.

The studies of breast screening with mammography are randomized controlled trials and were conducted in the UK, Europe, Scandinavia, and North America beginning in the 1960s. What they had in common was that they each had a control group—one group of women *were not* invited to screening and the study group of women *were* invited to screening. The women were assigned to the study or control groups randomly, so that the chances of women eventually getting cancer would be equal in the two groups. The outcome, measured many years later, was the number of women in each group who had died of breast cancer. If the number of women who died of breast cancer in the study group (those invited for a screening mammogram) was lower than the number of women who died of breast cancer in the control group it would mean that mammograms saved lives. The difference in the number of deaths in the groups had to be big enough to have not occurred just by chance. For example, if there were 10,000 women in each group, and after 15 years of follow-up the number of women in the study group that had died was 10 and the number in the control group was 12, that would not be a large enough difference to be meaningful. The technical expression is that it would not be *statistically significant*. However one has to look a little deeper to understand the studies better.

First, you may have noticed that most of the studies were based on an "invitation" to have a screening mammogram and not that the women in the study group actually had a screening mammogram. The control groups were not women who did not have a screening mammogram, but rather were women "not invited to screening." This is a subtle but very important detail.

In all of the studies, there were women who were invited, but never had a mammogram. Some came once, but not again. If one of these women developed cancer and died of it, her death would still be counted in the mammogram group, even if she never had a mammogram. The technical term for this is *non-compliance*.

In most of the trials, the women didn't know there was a study going on. The women in the control group just carried on as usual. Some of those women had mammograms, maybe got diagnosed with breast cancer and were treated. The technical term for women in the control group being screened is *contamination bias*.

In a study performed in Canada, the women were told that there was going to be a study, and they were asked to volunteer to participate. Many women showed up to volunteer. But unlike all the other trials, these women were first given a breast examination by a nurse, and then assigned to receive a mammogram (the study group) or not receive a mammogram (the control group). In other words, all the women had a screening breast physical examination by a trained nurse so that the study was really a test of adding mammograms to a skilled breast examination rather than a test of a population-based policy to invite women for screening mammograms.

One issue with the women being volunteers for the study is that many women who volunteered wanted to have a mammogram, and really wanted to be assigned to the mammogram group. Some of the women who were assigned to the control group (who weren't supposed to have mammograms) found a way to have a mammogram outside the trial. About one-quarter of the women in the control group actually had a mammogram and this would dilute the difference between the "mammogram" and "no mammogram" arms of the study. Another issue with the Canadian study is that the women tended to be well educated, fit, and have good access to health care services so that the breast cancer death rate was very low in both arms of the study. These issues, that all women had a physical examination, that a significant number of women in the control had a mammogram outside the study, and the "healthy volunteer effect" contributed to the Canadian trial not showing a difference in breast cancer death rates even though the women in the mammogram arm of the study were found to have more early cancers.

When the randomized controlled studies are evaluated together, they show an overall mortality reduction of 30%, even though non-compliance and contamination bias were occurring. It's therefore certain that if one were to consider only women who had a mammogram and compared them to women who didn't have a mammogram, the mortality difference would have been higher.

The chance of developing breast cancer (and therefore the value of screening mammograms) increases with age. A first mammogram will find approximately two cancers per 1000 women screened in their 40s, five cancers per 1000 women screened in their 50s and 10 cancers per 1000 women screened in their 70s. Screening mammograms can find cancers as small as a few millimetres in diameter and too small to feel. Women with such cancers have a much higher survival rate than women with cancers found when they are large enough to be felt by the woman or her doctor. As women age, other health problems play an increasing role in their lives. If a woman's life expectancy is less than 10 years, she is unlikely to benefit from the detection of a cancer before it can be felt.

How often should women have screening mammograms?

The question of how often women should have a mammogram also relates to the results of the randomized trials and how they were designed. Some of the studies screened women every year, some less often. Not surprisingly, there was a relationship between the length of time between screenings and the mortality reduction. In addition, mammograms are better able to detect small, curable cancers in women with fatty rather than dense breast tissue.

Breast cancer tends to grow faster in younger women. Age 50 is used as a surrogate (substitute) for the age of menopause and the definition of "younger" women in terms of breast screening policy. There is no abrupt change in the breast at age 50 and many women have not started menopause by age 50, so they should consider their breasts to be like those of younger women in terms of cancer exposure to hormones. Some women's breasts become less dense and composed of more fat as they age, but it's a gradual process. Women taking hormones for treatment of menopausal symptoms tend to have denser breasts, similar to premenopausal women. In a study from the Screening Mammography Program of British Columbia, women older than age 50 who had attended the program for an annual mammogram were compared to women who had mammograms about every 2 years. The cancers found at screening in women who came every 2 years were bigger, and more likely to have spread to their lymph nodes, than women who came every year. Survival after a diagnosis of breast cancer was similar at 5 years whether women had mammograms every year or every 2 years but was estimated to be 1% better at 10 years with annual mammograms. The women who had mammograms every year underwent substantially more diagnostic tests for abnormal mammograms that turned out not to be cancer. The bottom line is that women in their 50s and older should have a mammogram at least every 2 years. Younger women, those with dense breasts, those still menstruating, or those on hormone replacement therapy may benefit from annual mammograms. Doing mammograms at intervals beyond 3 years may miss finding a developing cancer while it is still small and highly curable.

What about younger or older women?

Some screening programs (for example, in British Columbia and the USA) invite women age 40 to 49 years to participate. Other programs require a doctor's referral at this age. Women younger than 40 years may benefit from screening if they are at very high risk on the basis of a family history with multiple breast or ovarian cancers, or if they had radiation therapy for Hodgkin's' lymphoma when they were younger. Mammogram screening before the age of 40 years should only be done after a careful discussion with an informed doctor (see Chapter 42). Women older than 79 years are increasingly likely to have other health problems simply because of their age. However, a woman in her 70s or 80s without any other health problems and who is likely to live another 10 years could benefit from continued breast screening.

Should women be taught breast self-examination?

Carefully conducted, large research studies have shown that women taught to perform breast self-examination (BSE) did not have smaller cancers and had no better chance of survival if they were diagnosed with breast cancer, compared to women who were not taught BSE. As a result, regular BSE is falling out of favour as a screening test. However, many women find the breast cancer themselves and although BSE is not proven to reduce mortality, women who choose to do it should be informed how to do it effectively.

All women have a degree of lumpiness and texture in their breasts, but no two women are exactly the same. It takes practice to learn what your own normal texture feels like, but once you know that, you're more likely to realize when there has been a change if a lump develops. For women who are still having menstrual periods, the best time to do BSE is just after the period. That is the time of the cycle when most women's breasts are the least lumpy and tender. Also, because breast texture varies through the month, doing BSE at the same phase of the cycle increases the chance that if you notice a change it may be due to some real change rather than hormonal variation through your cycle.

Women who have had a cancer of one breast are at risk of a recurrence in that breast and of developing cancer in the other breast. The risk of developing cancer in the other breast is approximately 3 to 5% over 10 years. Women with a previous breast cancer, therefore, may be particularly motivated to do BSE. For assistance in learning how to do BSE, ask your nurse or doctor at the cancer centre or contact the cancer information service in your area. In addition, for an illustration of a suggested BSE technique see the Appendix at the back of this book.

What are the limitations of screening?

Not all breast cancers can be found by a mammogram. Even more cancers are missed by breast self-examination. Failure to detect cancer may occur because the cancer is the same density as the woman's normal breast glands or the cancer is so far to the edge of the breast that it is missed by the mammogram. Approximately 25% of breast cancers in women age 40 to 49, 15% in women age 50 to 59, and 10% in women older than 60 will not be visible on a screening mammogram. For these women, even though a cancer is developing in the breast the mammogram is "negative." A concern with these "false negatives" is that they may lead to false reassurance. A woman could delay seeking medical help for a new lump if she has recently had a "negative" mammogram. Digital mammograms have been found to be more sensitive in detecting cancers in women younger than age 50 with dense breasts.

Another downside of screening is that many women have "false-positives." This means that the mammogram is reported to be "abnormal" when in fact no cancer is present. This can happen when there is a non-cancerous lump, like a cyst or fibroadenoma, benign calcification, or an area of normal tissue that looks a little prominent. False positives occur in 10 to 15% of woman on a first mammogram and 5 to 7% of women having a second or subsequent mammogram. The lower rate on repeat mammograms is because the radiologist has the first mammogram for comparison. Women with an abnormal test get understandably alarmed and will need to have additional tests to determine if the abnormality is cancer or a "false-positive." Many women find it very stressful to wait for the additional tests to be done. Overall, only 5% of women with an abnormal screening mammogram will turn out to have a breast cancer.

Some cancers are discovered by routine physical examinations by doctors or nurses. Compared to mammograms or women finding cancers themselves, relatively few breast cancers each year are detected this way. An annual examination with your family physician should include examination of both breasts, the lymph node areas in the axillae (armpits), and above the clavicles (collar bones). Any persistent or new lump or change in your breast should be investigated, even if a screening mammogram is "negative" or normal.

What about other tests for screening?

Mammography is the only screening test that has been proven to reduce deaths from breast cancer, because it is the only one that has been tested against a control group. Two other tests that have been tested (but not against a control group) are ultrasound and MRI.

Magnetic resonance imaging (MRI) has proven to be the most sensitive test in finding cancer, but it also finds even more abnormalities that are not cancer than mammography does. Furthermore, the cost of an MRI is much higher (up to 40 times more higher) than a mammogram and the MRI test requires an injection. Other issues with MRI are that most MRI machines have a weight limit, and cannot accommodate obese women, and most MRI units are "closed" so are not tolerated by women who are claustrophobic. Finally, if an abnormality is seen on the MRI, and a biopsy is required, it is much more difficult, time-consuming, and expensive to do a biopsy with MRI-guidance than it is for a biopsy with mammogram or ultrasound guidance. So MRI is not appropriate for screening women at average risk. Current recommendations for screening MRI are limited to women at very high risk of developing breast cancer such as women known to have an inherited mutation of the BRCA1 or BRCA2 gene (see Chapter 42).

Ultrasound is used frequently as a diagnostic test for women who have a lump or for women whose screening mammogram shows a lump. An ongoing large trial of ultrasound as a supplementary screening test to a mammogram is showing very good results for women who have dense breast tissue. Ultrasound is much less expensive than MRI, but not as sensitive. It allows guided needle biopsy of an abnormality, but like mammography and MRI, finds many abnormalities that are not cancer. It is more labour-intensive (time-consuming) to perform compared to a mammogram, and is not covered by medical insurance everywhere. It has been suggested that ultrasound in addition to mammograms be done for women with dense breasts and who are at higher than average risk, or for women who would otherwise qualify for MRI but who are obese or claustrophobic.

Thermography is a test that measures temperature in the breasts, and has been around since the 1970s. The theory is that cancers are hotter than normal breast tissue because tumours have a greater blood supply than normal tissues. Thermography can find big cancers that are usually palpable or visible (or both) with other tests such as mammograms and ultrasound. Thermography has not been proven to be successful at finding the small cancers that are the detection goal of a screening test and the false positive rate of thermography is unacceptably high.

Breast specific gamma imaging (BSGI) is a nuclear medicine test that is showing some promise in breast cancer screening in early research. It involves injecting radioactive material into an arm vein, and then imaging the breasts with a camera that measures the radioactivity in the breasts. It is showing good sensitivity and fewer false positives than some other tests, and it is less expensive than MRI. There is currently no method for doing guided needle biopsy of abnormalities seen on BSGI. Also, the radiation dose needs to be addressed. During a mammogram the dose of radiation is very small and is limited to the breasts. With BSGI the radioactivity is injected into a vein and the whole body is exposed to a low dose of radiation. More research on this promising test is needed.

SECTION FOUR

What do I do when I find a lump?

CHAPTER SEVEN

A *visit to the doctor*

Finding a lump or a new breast thickening

THE DISCOVERY OF A NEW BREAST LUMP or a change in one's breast such as a new thickening understandably causes tremendous anxiety. It may help to know that nearly 80% of lumps are benign (not cancerous). However, noticing a lump is often the first sign that may lead to a diagnosis of breast cancer. It is important to show any new lump or other breast abnormality to your doctor—and you should expect that it will be looked at in some detail.

What should happen when I show the lump to a doctor?

The doctor should ask when you first noticed the lump or thickening in the breast and whether it has changed, especially in relation to your menstrual cycle. Any previous breast problems and risk factors will be discussed, including biopsies, infections or injuries, and facts regarding your menstrual cycle, use of medications or hormones, and your family history (that is, whether breast cancer has occurred in family members).

It is best to examine the breasts of a premenopausal woman a week or two after the menstrual period, but if there is a worrisome lump you should not delay that first visit. During the breast examination you and the doctor are usually alone in the examining room, but you may request the presence of a nurse or bring a family member or friend along for moral support and as a "second set of ears" to help remember what has been said.

You will be asked to disrobe at least the upper half of your body. Depending on your physician's judgment, you may have a partial or complete physical examination. This may include listening to your chest and examining the lymph node areas in your neck and armpits, both breasts, and the abdomen. A pelvic examination is part of a yearly health exam and may be done, but it is not essential to the diagnosis of breast cancer.

What happens next?

Depending on what the doctor thinks about the abnormality you may need no further tests. The doctor's recommendation will depend partly on your age. Age greatly affects the chance that a lump will be breast cancer (see Chapter 3). If you are in your teens, a breast lump is almost certainly benign: breast cancer is very rare in this age group. If you are in your 20s, the vast majority of lumps are benign, but an occasional case of breast cancer is seen every year. In the 30s and 40s, breast cancer becomes more frequent, and among postmenopausal women there is a substantial possibility that a new breast lump will be from cancer.

Following the office visit and examination, you may be sent for a mammogram, ultrasound, or other tests. Assessment of your particular breast problem may require consultation with a surgeon, or you may need a biopsy, which involves removal of some tissue for further examination either with a small needle or by surgery (see Chapter 10). If there is a new lump a biopsy may be considered even if the mammogram and ultrasound are normal.

CHAPTER EIGHT

Breast lumps and other problems

Breast cysts

MANY WOMEN EXPERIENCE PAIN, lumpiness, and swelling of the breasts. Such women are often described as having *fibrocystic* disease. The tender, lumpy-feeling tissue may be completely normal, or may contain fluid-filled lumps called cysts. As a woman's hormones change through the menstrual cycle, the fluid-filled cysts may become intermittently enlarged and tender, especially in the days before a menstrual period begins.

As a rule, cysts do not turn into cancer. However, if a biopsy is done and the cells lining the cysts or ducts show excessive cell growth (hyperplasia) and an abnormal appearance under the microscope (atypia), there is a higher risk of breast cancer developing (see Chapter 2). Any new change in the breast, especially if it involves only one side, may be a sign of cancer and should be checked carefully by a doctor. Changes in the skin of the breast, such as redness or swelling in a woman who is not pregnant or breast-feeding, should be checked by a doctor. New breast redness should not be attributed to an infection unless the woman is breast-feeding. Otherwise a biopsy should be done.

Breast changes that may indicate cancer

Breast lumps

There is no absolute way to describe the feeling of a cancerous lump as compared to a non-cancerous (benign) lump. Some women say that they knew it was different from other lumps they had felt in the past. Cancer lumps are usually firm or hard. They are generally painless but may be tender or sore. Not all cancers are lumps—some appear as "thickenings" or "ridges" but generally, thickened areas are caused by benign changes. Sometimes women first notice a lump in the armpit—an enlarged lymph node. Lumps that feel as though they are attached to the skin or also have skin redness are especially likely to be cancerous.

Nipple changes

Crusting, ulceration, or eczema (weeping) of the nipple that does not go away in a few days may be the result of breast cancer cells growing into the nipple. This can be due to cancer or to another condition called Paget's disease in which cancer cells grow between the skin cells of the nipple (see Chapter 13). If the nipple becomes inverted (turns inward) it may be a sign of a growing cancer pulling on the ligaments of the breast as it enlarges.

Discharge from the nipple

A small amount of clear or whitish discharge can be squeezed from the nipple of most women and is *not* a cause for concern. If a discharge occurs on its own, spontaneously and is from a particular milk duct, it should be discussed with your doctor. If the discharge is bloody, it is usually due to a small, benign growth (a papilloma) in one of the milk ducts. However sometimes an early cancer may show up as bleeding or a brownish/rusty staining in the bra. A bleeding discharge should be investigated by your doctor and may require surgical removal of the bleeding milk duct.

Breast pain

Breast pain without a lump and without a worrisome abnormality on a mammogram or ultrasound is not a sign of cancer and, despite careful examination and follow-up, the cause is not usually found. Thankfully, the pain generally lessens over time. However, a new, persistent localized area of pain or pain associated with a lump should not be ignored in the mistaken belief that breast cancer is not painful.

Changing breast size and skin changes

Occasionally one breast may become larger or swollen. The skin or nipple may show dimpling, redness, or thickening. These changes are particularly worrisome because they could indicate that cancer has already spread to lymph nodes and is blocking the drainage of fluid from the breast. Changes in breast size or skin changes should be investigated carefully as they may be associated with a cancer.

Enlarged nodes or lumps in the armpit

Some breast cancers are first diagnosed as a lump in the armpit. Lymph nodes in the armpit (axilla) may become swollen from causes other than cancer such as an infection, but a new lump in the armpit should be investigated with a mammogram, ultrasound, sometimes a breast MRI, and a biopsy of the lymph node.

CHAPTER NINE

Diagnostic mammograms, ultrasounds, MRI scans, and PET scans

Diagnostic mammograms

A MAMMOGRAM IS A LOW-DOSE X-RAY of the breast. When a new lump is found, a diagnostic mammogram should be performed on *both* breasts. This allows evaluation of the lump, a check of the rest of that breast, and an assessment of the opposite breast for unsuspected abnormalities. Each breast is flattened or compressed first from top-to-bottom and then diagonally from side-to-side, between the plastic plates of the mammogram machine as shown in Figure 7. If there is a lump that you feel, the technologist may ask you to show it to her so she can mark it on a diagram. She may also put a sticker on it. The sticker has a tiny piece of lead on it, which will show on the mammogram as a bright white dot, so the radiologist will know where the lump was located. Additional magnification and compression views may be taken to highlight parts of the breast that look abnormal or were not seen completely in the standard views. For example, an image may be taken to focus on the extreme outside part of the breast or if there appears to be a localized lump. Some apparent "lumps" are due to overlapping of gland areas in the breast. With additional localized compression, the area is spread out and the "lump" may disappear, proving that it is not cancer.

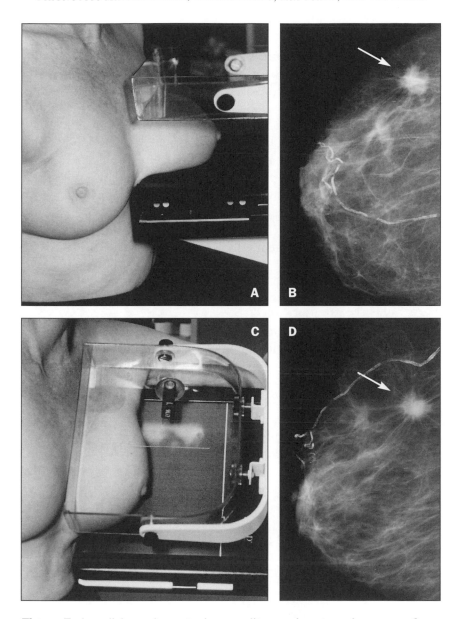

Figure 7: Localizing a breast abnormality requires two views, one from the top and one from the side of the breast. When the mammogram is taken with the breast flat (panel A) the X-rays pass from top to bottom through the breast to produce the image in panel B. X-rays passing from side-to-side though the breast (panel C) produce the image in panel D. The arrow identifies the cancer on panels B and D.

Signs of cancer on a mammogram

There is no single feature on a mammogram that always indicates cancer. However, there are features that are suggestive of cancer: a lump with jagged edges, clusters of irregular, tiny, white dots that indicate calcium deposits, a pattern of tissue that looks like spokes on a wheel, and thickening of the overlying skin.

There are several possible reasons, other than cancer, for lumps or calcium deposits on a mammogram. If a lump or calcium deposit is very smooth and round or unchanged for several years, it is probably not cancer and doesn't need to be biopsied. However, if an abnormality is new or irregular, it may require biopsy to check if a cancer is present. Therefore, expert interpretation is necessary before a biopsy is recommended.

Other information from the mammogram

How big is the lump or cancer?

The mammogram can give information about the size of the lump or cancer. Calcifications, for instance, can sometimes be seen to extend many centimetres from the lump that you feel. If the lump turns out to be cancer, this information will be relevant in deciding whether a mastectomy is necessary or whether it is feasible to save the breast. It is important, therefore, to have a mammogram to obtain this information before a biopsy is done because the breast may feel too bruised or sore to obtain a mammogram after the biopsy. Also, the bruise from a biopsy may cause confusion reading the mammogram: it can make a non-cancerous lump look suspicious.

Is there another "hidden" cancer?

If one cancer is found, it is important to also check the rest of the breast and the breast on the opposite side to make sure that an additional hidden (occult) cancer is not missed. One or two women in 100 who are diagnosed with a breast cancer will be found to have a cancer in the other breast at the same time.

Are there different kinds of mammograms?

Some mammogram machines use X-ray film to record the image, and other machines use digital detectors to sense the X-rays coming through the breast and project the digital image onto a computer screen. It is known that overall, film and digital mammograms are equally good at finding cancers but digital mammograms can be more sensitive for the detection of cancer in women with dense breasts, such as those women under the age of 50 years. There are other advantages of digital mammography. The image is stored on the computer, unlimited copies can be generated, and the image cannot be misplaced like a piece of film. Also, if the picture is over or under-exposed, it can be adjusted on the computer screen, like a picture taken with a digital camera, so there is less need for the technologist to repeat the X-ray. Digital mammography machines may be used for either diagnostic or screening mammograms. Gradually all clinics will be converting to digital mammograms.

Screening mammograms (see Chapter 6) are generally two views of each breast and are done in healthy women with no apparent abnormality in their breasts. The goal of a screening mammogram is to detect a small, early breast cancer before it can be felt. *Diagnostic mammograms* are done to closely examine an abnormality found during screening or for women who have a new lump or change in the breast. A diagnostic mammogram starts with the same pictures as a screening mammogram: two views per breast. Extra views may be taken of the area of concern, including magnified views to more clearly define the area and decide if it looks sufficiently normal that a recheck in 6 months is recommended, or whether it would be better to do a biopsy. If the radiologist feels there is a less than 2% chance of an abnormality being cancer, then a biopsy is not recommended and the woman is asked to return for another mammogram in 6 months to confirm that the abnormality is not changing.

Mammograms do not show all cancers, but if they are done properly and read by an experienced radiologist, the majority of cancers are visible.

Ultrasound

A mammogram can show a lump but it cannot tell if the lump is a solid cancer, a solid benign (non-cancerous) tumour (such as a fibroadenoma), or a cyst (fluid filled cavity—which is usually benign). An ultrasound may be helpful in determining if a lump is a cyst or a solid mass. Ultrasound uses sound waves rather than

X-rays to assess the breast.

The ultrasound machine includes a small hand-held device that is pressed against the skin while sound waves are transmitted painlessly through the breast. Gel is put on the skin to better transmit the sound waves through the skin surface. The sound waves are transmitted through the breast tissue and bounce off structures in the body, back to the ultrasound receiver. A computer receiving the signals then converts the pattern of rebounding sound waves into images that appear on a computer monitor.

What does an ultrasound show?

The main purpose of an ultrasound is to find out if a lump in the breast is solid (composed of tissue), or a cyst (filled with fluid). If a lump meets the strict criteria for a simple cyst, we can be 100% confident that it is *not* cancer. Cysts are the most common lumps in the breast. They do not turn into cancer, and women with cysts are at no higher risk of developing breast cancer than women who do not have cysts. Women who get cysts tend to get more cysts as they get older, but cysts in the breasts are not related to having cysts elsewhere in the body (ovaries, kidneys, etc.). Cysts can stay the same size or they can disappear without treatment. Sometimes they fluctuate in size with the menstrual cycle: they can feel bigger, harder, and sore before a period, and then smaller, softer, and less sore after a period. If a cyst gets big and sore, it can be drained with a thin needle (smaller than the needles used to take a blood test), but cysts that have been drained come back about 30% of the time, If a cyst is not bothering the woman, it can safely be left alone.

Not all cysts look completely typical on an ultrasound. This can happen if a cyst is in the process of shrinking, and the fluid in it is thicker and less watery. If the radiologist feels that this is probably the case he or she may suggest a repeat ultrasound in 6 months, or may offer to drain it. If a cyst is partly solid, a needle biopsy may be done (see Chapter 10).

An ultrasound may also show that a lump is solid. Most solid lumps are not cancer, although this varies with the age of the woman. If a lump is solid but looks exactly like a typical fibroadenoma (the most common non-cancerous solid lump), the radiologist may recommend repeat ultrasound in 6 months. They only do so if they are more than 98% sure that it's *not* a cancer. If the radiologist is less

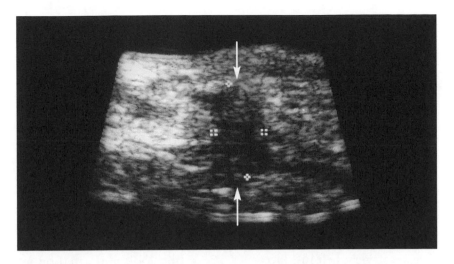

Figure 8: This ultrasound shows the characteristic "taller-than-wide" orientation of a cancer (between the white arrows). Not all cancers are taller than they are wide, but virtually all masses with this appearance are cancer.

than 98% sure they should recommend a core biopsy (see below).

Cancers are usually solid and have an irregular outline. The clues on the ultrasound that virtually always indicates that a lump is cancer are when the mass looks "taller than wide" (Figure 8), or when it has jagged edges.

Ultrasound can also be used to direct a needle into a breast lump so that fluid, cells, or small pieces of tissue can be removed and examined under the microscope. This is called an *ultrasound-guided needle biopsy*. When ultrasound guidance is used to position the needle, the placement is more precise than when the needle is placed by finger guidance alone, especially if the lump is deep in the breast. When using ultrasound guidance, a negative or non-diagnostic result is virtually equivalent to a diagnosis of "not cancer." However, if there is a persistent, suspicious mass on the mammogram or ultrasound, it should be removed surgically, even if the needle test does not find any cancer cells. Part of the job of the radiologist who does the needle test is to decide whether the result on the pathology report explains and matches the impression from looking at the ultrasound (and/or mammogram picture).

If the picture was suspicious of cancer, and the pathology is not cancer, the "better-safe-than-sorry" recommendation is to surgically remove the abnormality. This is usually a small operation done with local anaesthetic (freezing).

Magnetic resonance imaging (MRI)

Magnetic resonance imaging (MRI) gives a different type of picture than a mammogram or ultrasound and there is no radiation involved. An MRI uses a powerful magnet and a radiofrequency coil to create images before and after the intravenous injection of a material (gadolinium) that makes small cancers (and some non-cancerous tissue) become more easily visible. MRI has a very high sensitivity, even in dense breasts where mammograms are sometimes not very helpful. However, areas that look abnormal on an MRI are frequently not cancer. Many normal areas may appear abnormal on an MRI. A specially trained radiologist can often tell the difference between benign and cancerous changes, but still, approximately 25% of women who do *not* have breast cancer will have something abnormal reported on a breast MRI scan. This can lead to concern that cancer may be present and may prompt additional tests, including biopsies.

Studies have shown that MRI screening is helpful for women who carry an inherited mutation that predisposes them to develop breast cancer. Such women have a very high risk of developing breast cancer (see Chapter 42) and may benefit from regular breast screening with MRI in addition to mammograms. However, routine MRI screening of the general population, without inherited mutations, is not recommended.

MRI may also be helpful in diagnosis when the mammogram and ultrasound do not provide enough information, such as when the cancer first shows up in an axillary (armpit) lymph node with no disease found in the breast or after surgery when questions arise about whether all the cancer was removed. MRI is also useful in other situations such as monitoring the response to therapy of locally advanced cancer or in follow-up after lumpectomy plus radiation therapy when there are unusual changes in the breast scar.

Positron emission tomography scans

Positron emission tomography (PET) uses a small dose of radio-active-labeled glucose (sugar) to create an image of the extent of cancer in the body. This can sometimes be helpful in telling how far the cancer has spread. A small dose of radioactive glucose is injected into a vein and the scan is taken a short time later. Cells in the body that have a high metabolic activity (growing rapidly or consuming a lot of energy) concentrate the glucose and show up as a bright spot on the scan. Many invasive cancers are rapidly growing compared to their surrounding tissues and show up as "hot" on the PET scan. If the cancer has spread to lymph nodes or other organs such as the lung, bone, or liver, the PET scan may show "hot spots" in these other organs. However, to be visible on a PET scan, the cancer lump generally has to be larger than half a centimetre (1/4 inch). Small microscopic clusters or individual cancer cells do not show up on a PET scan. Also, not all cancers, even when large, show up on a PET scan. Low grade, slow growing cancers are especially likely to result in a "negative" PET scan.

Research is being done with different types of injectable substances and specific types of breast cancer to understand how this powerful imaging technique can best be used in breast cancer. Machines that combine CT and PET are being used to more accurately localize actively dividing cancer within the body.

CHAPTER TEN

Biopsies

What is a biopsy and when is it needed?

IN MANY CASES, MAMMOGRAMS AND ULTRASOUND (see Chapter 9) give enough information to diagnose a benign condition in the breast and no further tests are necessary. However, if the diagnosis is still uncertain, then the next step is to take some breast tissue from the area and look at it under a microscope. The process of removing the cells or tissue is called "performing a biopsy." There are several ways to do this, most of which are quick and relatively painless.

A fine needle biopsy

A fine needle biopsy (or fine-needle aspiration biopsy) can be done in the doctor's office. It takes only a few seconds and usually causes no more pain than having a blood test. The skin may or may not be frozen with a local anaesthetic. Then, while holding the lump between two fingers, the surgeon or pathologist uses a syringe with a very thin needle to draw out some material from the lump (Figure 9). A fine-needle biopsy may also be done by a radiologist using ultrasound to ensure that the needle is accurately positioned in the lump, especially if the abnormal area cannot be felt.

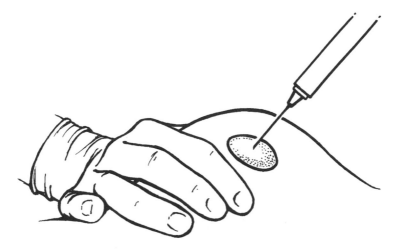

Figure 9: A needle biopsy involves the use of a needle to remove some material from the lump. The needle can be directed into the lump by feel or with ultrasound guidance (see Chapter 9).

If the lump is a cyst

If the lump is a cyst, the fluid in the cyst will be drawn into the syringe and the lump will disappear. No further action may be necessary. The cyst fluid may be a wide range of colours: anything from a pale clear yellow to a thick, dark inky green. Since little information can be obtained from this fluid, it is usually discarded. If the cyst fluid is bloody or if the lump remains even after all the fluid has been drained, there is cause for concern. In these cases, additional investigation is needed because there may be a cancer that is producing the cyst fluid or the lump. A surgical biopsy may be recommended. Also, if a cyst feels benign but keeps coming back after several finger-guided aspirations, an ultrasound is advisable to determine if there is a solid component that needs to be sampled.

If the lump is solid

If the lump is solid, small clumps of cells (invisible to the naked eye) will be drawn into the needle. These cells are smeared onto slides or added to a jar with fluid and then prepared for the microscope. The preparation and interpretation of the slides may take a few days.

Based on a microscopic examination of the cells a report will be issued that the aspiration was either "positive," "negative" or "non-diagnostic." If the report is "positive for cancer," the diagnosis is correct over 95% of the time. If the report is "negative for cancer" or "non-diagnostic," the lesion is usually benign, but as with any test, there could be false negative results. This could happen because the needle missed the cancer, or because the cancer cells, although present, were not removed during that aspiration. A non-diagnostic test could mean that no breast cells were obtained by the needle aspiration. A non-diagnostic test must be evaluated within the context of the physical examination and breast imaging. Sometimes it is necessary to repeat the fine needle biopsy or obtain larger amounts of tissue with a core biopsy (see next paragraph) or a surgical biopsy. On some occasions the aspirate may contain only fat cells. If the doctor who did the needle biopsy thought that the area was likely to be a ridge or nodule of breast fat and fat is in fact detected in the fine needle biopsy, then no surgical follow-up is needed. This can only be determined by the physician who has done the aspiration and after it is reviewed with the context of what the examiner felt and saw on the breast imaging. If the needle aspiration pathology, the physical examination and breast imaging are all benign, then it is rare that the abnormal area is cancer. But, if any one of the tests is suspicious for cancer, then further testing and removal of the lump may be indicated.

A core biopsy

For a core biopsy, a special needle is used to obtain multiple small cores of tissue. There are two kinds of core biopsy: a spring core, that makes a loud snap sound, and a vacuum core, that makes a whirring sound. Your doctor will probably let you hear the sound before the biopsy is done, so you know what to expect, and so it doesn't startle you when you hear it during the test. These needles are wider than a fine-needle, but after local anaesthetic is given, the needle feels virtually the same as the smaller needle. The freezing medicine takes away the sharp needle sensation, but you will still have the sensations of touch and dull pressure.

The spring core biopsy needle works by using a spring to advance the needle into an abnormal area to cut small slivers of tissue, similar in size to flakes of coconut. After the local anaesthetic is injected, a small "nick" is made in the skin, about half the length of a grain of rice, and the needle is inserted into the breast. When the samples are obtained, the spring makes a loud snapping sound like a stapler. Core biopsies are usually performed using ultra-sound or mammographic guidance. For ultrasound guidance, the radiologist will be scanning while the needle is inserted to ensure that the needle goes into the lump. Using mammographic guidance requires a special machine called a stereotactic unit attached to the mammogram machine and a special device to do the core-needle biopsy. Some stereotactic units are designed for the patient to lie on her stomach with her breast protruding through a hole in the table. Others have the patient seated or lying on her side. Core biopsies are being used increasingly frequently, as they reduce the number of unnecessary surgical biopsies and help in more accu-rate planning for the final surgery. A technique using a vacuum or other suction device attached to the core needle biopsy equipment allows larger areas of the breast to be removed without leaving a surgical scar. Often special non-reactive clips are inserted into the breast to mark the area of the biopsy in case a surgical biopsy may be needed afterward. These clips are not harmful and can stay in your breast if necessary.

A surgical (open) biopsy

A surgical biopsy (also called an *open biopsy*) involves making a small cut or incision in the skin of the breast and cutting out a piece of breast tissue (Figure 10). This usually takes place in a hos-pital, and can be done under a local or general anaesthetic. Most patients today are diagnosed with an initial core needle biopsy rather than an open biopsy, but in circumstances where a breast abnormality is not suitable for needle biopsy, an open biopsy may still be required.

Excisional biopsy: the whole lump is taken out

In addition to removing the entire lump, a small rim of the sur-rounding normal breast tissue is also removed. This leaves a small scar, but unless the lump was large relative to the size of the breast, it should not form a defect in the shape of the breast. Although such a biopsy can be a frightening experience, it is actually quite a simple surgical procedure.

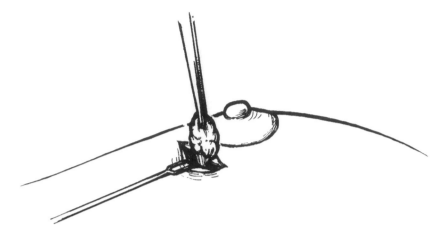

Figure 10: An open biopsy involves making a small cut in the skin and cutting out a piece of breast tissue.

Image-guided excisional biopsy

In this type of surgical biopsy the problem area within the breast is removed but, because the surgeon cannot feel the area, a type of guidance system, usually using a wire inserted through the skin prior to the surgery, is needed. The wire is usually placed by a radiologist using ultrasound, mammography, or possibly even an MRI to guide the placement of a small, thin, hooked wire into the problem area. The surgeon will use this wire to help guide the excision. In this manner, the lesion can be targeted with less chance of taking excess normal tissue.

For most abnormalities that are seen on a screening mammogram, a core biopsy is first recommended. If the results of the core biopsy suggest that the abnormal area should be removed surgically then this type of wire guidance is usually used. For example, if a small cancer that cannot be felt were diagnosed within the breast, a wire placed under breast imaging guidance would be used to help the surgeon find the cancer and remove it as a lumpectomy.

Incisional biopsy: only a part of the lump is removed

Using anaesthetic, the surgeon makes an incision through the skin and removes only a small part of the lump rather than the whole thing. This is done only when a lump is very large and when an excisional biopsy would cause a severe breast deformity or would not remove all of the cancer anyway. For example, when a cancer has invaded the skin or the chest wall, the doctor may do an incisional biopsy or core biopsy to confirm the diagnosis of cancer and obtain tissue for estrogen receptor and HER2 testing before discussing treatment options.

Other considerations

Generally, most suspicious masses should have a core needle biopsy as the first step to obtain tissue for diagnosis. Although in the past, women with an abnormality on their mammogram would have surgery to find out if it was cancer, core biopsy is so accurate, that now, women whose abnormalities are diagnosed as non-cancerous can be spared unnecessary surgery. When a core biopsy confirms cancer, the woman can have a single surgery to remove the cancer with clear margins.

If the lump needs to be removed for diagnosis using an open biopsy, it should be performed by a surgeon experienced in breast cancer surgery. The advantage is that the surgeon can assess the breast carefully and plan the position of the biopsy scar in such a way that it will fit with any additional surgery. The incision should always be placed to give the best cosmetic result and to make as little change in the shape of the breast as possible. The length of the biopsy scar will depend on the size of the lump, but it should not be more than a few centimetres long.

Whichever type of biopsy is done, the specimen is sent directly to the pathologist for a number of studies (see Chapter 12).

A *frozen section biopsy*

In some situations a quick decision must be made about treatment while in the operating room, and a "frozen section" or "quick section" is done. This means that a piece of breast tissue is frozen while the patient is still on the operating table and ultra-thin slices of the tissue are examined under the microscope. This takes about 10 to 20 minutes. The problem with this method is that it is neither as good nor as complete as the diagnosis made when the pathologist has more time to examine the entire tissue sample and look at sections from several different areas of the tissue. The diagnosis of cancer inside the milk ducts (called *in situ* cancer) can be especially difficult to make on a frozen section. Frozen sections are not performed as frequently today as they were in the past. The only reason to do a frozen section would be if the result found by the pathologist was going to have an immediate impact on the operation.

In cases where a diagnosis of cancer has not been made before the operation, it is usually best to perform the surgical biopsy and then wait for the pathologist to give a definite diagnosis, even if this takes a few days. Then, decisions about further tests and treatment can be made when the patient is awake and fully able to participate.

CHAPTER ELEVEN

If the screening mammogram is abnormal

What happens if my screening mammogram is abnormal?

IF YOU ARE TOLD that your screening mammogram is abnormal do *not* assume that you have cancer! An abnormal result simply means that you need further evaluation to find out if the abnormality is really a cancer or some other problem such as scarring or cysts.

The first step depends on the standard practice in your area. Some regions have adopted the approach where the woman is called back by the radiology clinic directly for additional mammogram or ultrasound examinations. Sometimes, all it takes is an additional mammogram picture to know that everything is fine. Sometimes an ultrasound is done. If a biopsy is performed, the pathology result is sent to your doctor. The radiologist will report to your doctor and make a follow-up recommendation. In some cases no follow-up is needed, and you can continue with regular screening. Other times, a 6-month follow-up examination will be suggested, and the radiologist will specify whether it should be a mammogram, an ultrasound, or both. If there is still concern, even if the needle biopsy shows no cancer, a surgical biopsy will be recommended.

In other regions the step after an abnormal screen is to see your family doctor to have a physical examination and to allow the family doctor to then organize additional tests. You will still need to have the extra mammograms or ultrasound (or both) as described above. Although some women would prefer to see their family doctor before the extra tests, often he or she cannot tell them much before the tests are done. As a result, many screening programs have adopted a direct recall system when the screening mammogram is abnormal.

A radiologist should compare the new mammogram to other mammograms you may have had previously. If it was the first time you had a mammogram in a new office, inform the technologist where you had your previous mammogram(s). Better yet would be to get the previous mammograms yourself and bring them to the new appointment.

A mass that has been present and unchanged for many years does not need to be biopsied. Often, more mammograms will be taken to provide greater detail of the abnormality (see Chapter 9). An ultrasound may be used to distinguish between a cyst and a solid mass. Also, a fine-needle or core biopsy done under ultrasound guidance or stereotactic control may provide more information (see Chapter 10).

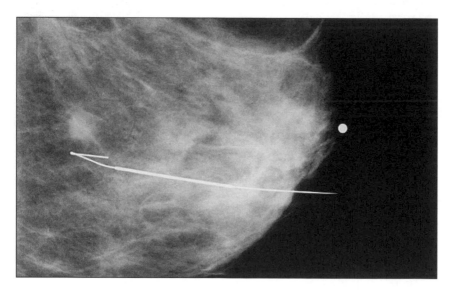

Figure 11: Guided by the mammogram, a fine wire with a hook on the end is placed through a needle into the vicinity of the suspicious area. At this stage the woman goes to the operating room for a biopsy.

Fine-wire localization biopsy

If the abnormality in your breast has been diagnosed as a cancer on the needle biopsy, or if it is still questionable after investigations have been done, it will have to be removed by surgical (open) biopsy so it can be examined in more detail. If the abnormality is too small to be felt by the surgeon, a technique called *fine-wire localization* is used to help the surgeon find the exact location of the abnormality in the breast.

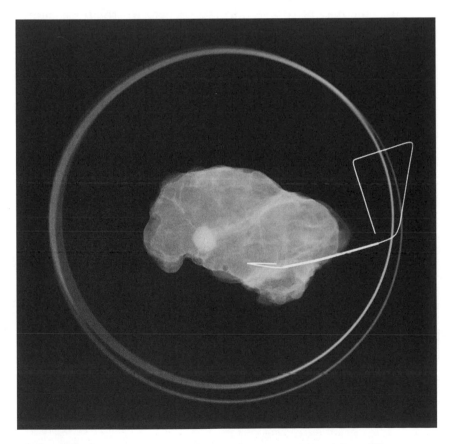

Figure 12: An X-ray of the biopsy specimen removed from the woman in Figure 11. The surgeon cut down along the wire until she reached the tip. She then removed the abnormal area and a margin of surrounding breast tissue. The abnormality turned out to be a 1 cm invasive ductal carcinoma; this procedure has an excellent chance for cure.

Before the surgery another mammogram or ultrasound is taken. With the breast held between the mammographic plates or using the ultrasound for guidance, the radiologist locates the abnormality and then gives local anaesthetic to freeze the skin. A thin needle is inserted into the breast and into the abnormal area. Then a very fine wire with a tiny hook on the end is threaded through the hollow needle and the needle is withdrawn, leaving the tiny hook at the end of the wire snagged near the suspicious area. The other end of the fine wire is sticking out of the skin (Figure 11). The wire is very thin, and can be folded against the skin and covered with a dressing. The patient is then taken to surgery for the open biopsy and the surgeon can follow the wire to find the area that needs to be removed. Depending on the type of abnormality that prompted the biopsy and the technique used to insert the fine wire, an X-ray or ultrasound of the biopsy specimen may be done to confirm that the suspicious area has been removed (Figure 12).

What type of cancer is it?

CHAPTER TWELVE

The pathology report:
Reading the cancer's telltale signs

WHEN A SURGEON REMOVES a suspicious lump from the breast or
a radiologist obtains a core needle biopsy, a lot of important information can be gained by looking at the removed tissue under the
microscope (Figures 13 and 14). A detailed microscopic examination
establishes whether cancer is present. In addition, the examination
provides information that helps predict how the cancer is likely to
behave. Is it likely to grow back? Where? When? With this information, a treatment strategy can be planned with the goal of preventing
recurrence and maximizing your chance of being cured. Uncovering
this information and reporting it is the role of the pathologist—a
physician specializing in the study of tissues. The pathologist's written summary is called the pathology report.

The three sections of the pathology report

The pathology report contains three main sections: the gross description of the tissues (as seen with the naked eye), the microscopic
description, and the summary (final diagnosis).

The gross description of the tissues

The pathologist reports on what he or she can see with the naked
eye: for instance the size of the lump, the number and size of any
lymph nodes and how close the cancer is to the edge of the specimen.

71

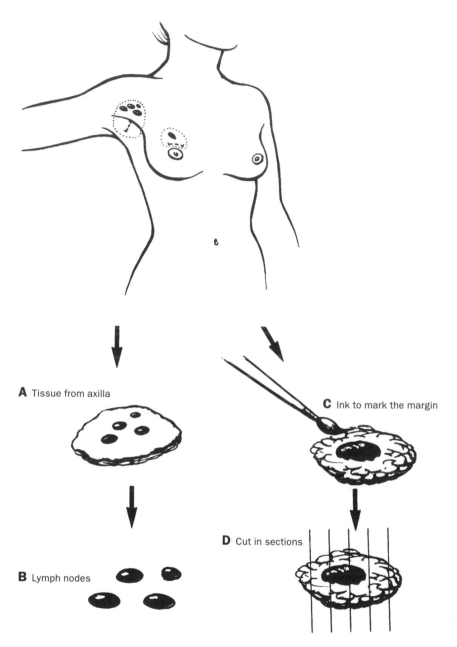

Figure 13: Tissue from the axillary dissection (A) is examined and any lymph nodes are removed and counted (B). The external surface of the breast tissue containing the cancer is painted with ink (C) and then the specimen is cut into sections (D).

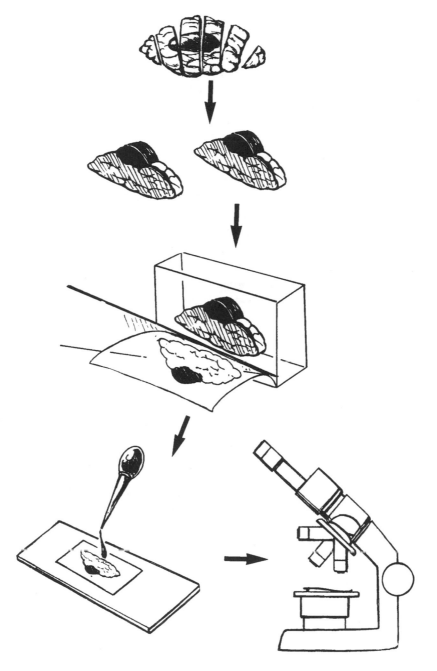

Figure 14: Preparation of a small piece of the breast lump for viewing on a microscope slide.

This is important: if the cancer is right against the edge rather than being centred within a block of normal-looking tissue, there is a higher likelihood that some cancer cells may have been left behind in the breast. Once samples are cut for microscopic examination, the rest of the excised tissue is immersed in a container of formaldehyde and labeled with your name. Specimens are stored like this for many years in case further examination is required.

The microscopic description

Under the microscope, breast cancer cells look different from normal cells. The pathologist will describe details of the type of cancer, the grade (an assessment of how abnormal or aggressive the cancer cells look), the number of mitoses—cells that have been "caught in the act" of multiplying, which is an indicator of the cancer's growth rate—and whether the cancer has invaded the tissues surrounding the main cancer, especially whether cancer cells are seen within the lymphatic or blood vessels in the breast. The report should also describe the amount of estrogen and progesterone receptor content in the cancer cells and the amount of activity (expression) of the HER2 gene (human epidermal receptor 2; also written as *her2-neu* or *c-erb-B2*). Over-expression of the HER2 gene increases the risk that the cancer will recur and also determines if the drug Herceptin will be useful (see Chapter 30).

If any lymph nodes have been removed from under the arm the pathologist will report on whether the cancer has spread into the lymph nodes. The pathology report should document how many nodes were found, and how many, if any, were affected by cancer, as well as the size of the involved lymph nodes. It should also mention whether the cancer has grown through the lymph node and out into the surrounding fat (called *extranodal* or *extracapsular extension*).

Final diagnosis

The pathologist's final diagnosis is a summary of the results of the gross and microscopic examinations. The process of tissue inspection and preparation of the report usually takes from 2 to 7 days. The report then becomes a permanent part of the patient's medical record. The important features that help predict the prognosis of the cancer and influence your doctor's recommendations about treatment are listed in Table 4.

Table 4	**Features of the pathology report that affect prognosis and treatment strategy**

The tumour

Size: measured in centimetres

Type: in situ, invasive, or mixed; ductal, lobular, or other (see Chapters 13 and 14)

Invasion: of the lymphatic or vascular spaces

Grade: the degree of aggressiveness, includes assessment of the number of mitoses (dividing cells), the appearance of the cell nuclei, and whether the cells are trying to form milk ducts

Necrosis (dying cells): a measure of the cancer's growth rate

Receptors: for estrogen and progesterone and the level of the receptor expression

HER2 status: presence or absence of gene overexpression

Extension of tumour: to skin, to muscle, to excision margins

Other prognostic markers: Ki67 (a measure of the grade of the tumour), p53, ploidy, p27, oncogenes, other growth factors may be reported but are not standard

The lymph nodes

Total number of lymph nodes recovered

Number of involved nodes

Maximum size of involved nodes

Extranodal extension (growth beyond the lymph nodes): present or absent

CHAPTER THIRTEEN

In situ cancer:
Cancer that has not invaded or spread

IN SITU CANCER IN THE BREAST refers to a cancer that is still within the milk ducts, the milk glands, or both. In other words, the cancer cells have not invaded through the walls of the milk ducts. The cancer cells are in the same place (or situation) where they first formed.

Ductal carcinoma in situ

As cancer cells accumulate inside a milk duct it may become blocked and enlarged (Figure 15). This is called *ductal carcinoma in situ* (DCIS) and is also referred to as *intraductal cancer*. Calcium tends to collect in the blocked ducts (Figure 16) and is visible on mammograms as tiny white lines and dots (Figure 17). These clusters of fine, irregular calcifications on a mammogram often indicate in situ cancer and, if present, a biopsy should be done. In situ cancer of the ducts accounts for 15 to 20% of the cancers found on screening mammograms. Ductal carcinoma in situ, if left untreated, may progress to form an invasive cancer with the potential for spreading throughout the body (Figure 16). The progression from in situ to invasive cancer can take as long as 5 to 10 years. If an invasive cancer is diagnosed after an area of DCIS is excised from the breast, the invasive cancer is most often found in the vicinity of the initial DCIS. This means that treatment for DCIS needs to concentrate on removing or killing all the abnormal

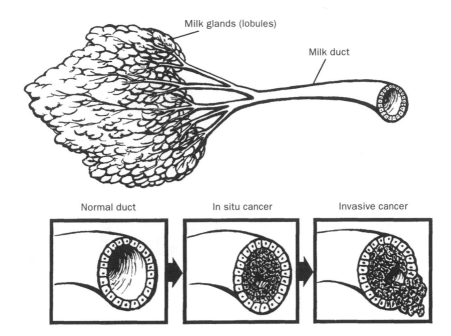

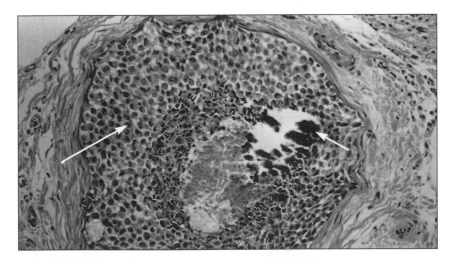

Figure 15: Cross-sectional view of milk duct. The duct may become filled with in situ cancer cells that eventually form an invasive cancer.

Figure 16: Ductal carcinoma in situ cells (large arrow) seen under the microscope. The dark material (small arrow) is a calcium deposit that has formed in an area of dead and dying cancer cells (necrosis).

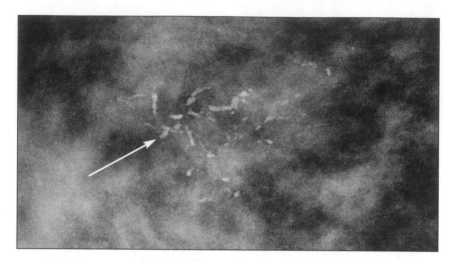

Figure 17: Calcium deposits typical of ductal carcinoma in situ as seen on a mammogram.

cells in the local area of the breast.

Ductal carcinoma in situ occurs as two different cell types, with one tending to progress to invasion more slowly than the other. The first type, which progresses more slowly, consists of smaller, more normal-looking cells. These cells may form solid, papillary, or cribiform types of DCIS. The second type, called *comedocarcinoma*, often progresses to invasion early in its growth and consists of large, irregularly shaped cells. Because they are growing quickly, these cells tend to outgrow their supply of sugar and oxygen. As a result, cells in the middle of the ducts start to die (called *necrosis*) and eventually the body deposits calcium in the dead cells (Figure 17). In many patients the DCIS may have both comedo-type and non-comedo-type growth patterns. Ductal carcinoma in situ may be estrogen receptor positive or negative (see Chapter 14). Chapter 23 describes the treatment of in situ cancers.

Lobular carcinoma in situ

Lobular carcinoma in situ (LCIS) refers to cancer cells that have formed in the milk glands (called *lobules*) and are still confined there. This type of in situ cancer is most often found in women around the age of menopause. Lobular carcinoma in situ is almost always hormonally responsive. The presence of LCIS carries a different significance compared to DCIS. While DCIS is a problem of the particular portion of the breast affected, with LCIS there is a higher risk of subsequent invasive breast cancer throughout the entire tissue of both breasts. Therefore, treatment of lobular carcinoma in situ (see Chapter 23) must be aimed at both breasts rather than just the affected one.

Paget's disease

Paget's disease is a rare form of in situ cancer that can occur in a "pure" form but is often accompanied by an invasive cancer. Paget's disease appears as a reddish, itching, scaling, or "eczema" of the nipple or areola caused by cancer cells in the skin of the nipple and areola. Although the traditional treatment is mastectomy, it may be possible to save the breast if there is no underlying invasive cancer. To save the breast it should be large enough to tolerate the removal of the skin surrounding the nipple and areola and the woman needs to accept that there will be a change in sensation and appearance due to the removal of the nipple and areola.

As well as removing the nipple and some surrounding skin, a sample of the breast tissue beneath should also be taken to make sure there is no accompanying invasive cancer. It is not yet clear whether radiation therapy should always follow surgical excision of Paget's disease, but in most cases, radiation treatment is added when using a breast-conserving approach to reduce the chance of cancer regrowth in the breast.

CHAPTER FOURTEEN

The different types of invasive cancer

What is invasive cancer?

CANCER CELLS HAVE TWO CHARACTERISTICS that are important. One is that the cells can grow through the walls of the milk ducts and glands and invade into the normal fatty tissue of the breast (Figure 15, page 77). As the cells grow in the fatty tissue they form a lump or thickening.

The second characteristic is that the invasive cancer cells can travel through the blood stream or lymphatic system. It is this ability to invade and spread through the body that makes us fear cancer. When cancer spreads to other parts of the body, we say it has *metastasized* and the tumours growing in areas away from the breast are called *metastases*. If we look at these metastases under the microscope, we would see that wherever they are in the body, they are actually breast cancer cells with features of a cancer that initially developed in the breast.

Invasive cancers do not usually grow like an expanding balloon. Rather, finger-like projections of cells grow out into the normal breast tissue from the main cancer. These finger-like projections may be seen under a microscope and sometimes even on a mammogram. Figure 7 (page 51) shows the typical appearance of an invasive cancer on a mammogram.

To determine how a cancer will behave in the future, the pathologist carefully assesses the tumour. Currently, cancers are divided into types according to their appearance under the microscope (the tumour histology). Using this classification, the classically recognized types of breast cancer are:

From ducts and glands
Infiltrating ductal carcinoma
– Type not otherwise specified (75%)
  – tubular (1%)
  – mucinous (1%)
  – colloid (1%)
  – medullary (1%)
  – inflammatory (3 to 5%)
Lobular carcinoma (15%)
Squamous carcinomas (less than 1%)
Mixed carcinomas (adenosquamous and
  metaplastic cancers) (less than 1%)

From other parts of the breast
Cystosarcoma phylloides (1%)
Sarcomas (less than 1%)
Lymphomas (less than 1%)

Ductal carcinoma, also called *mammary carcinoma* or *infiltrating ductal adenocarcinoma*, is the most common type of breast cancer. Lobular carcinomas, which account for about 15% of breast cancers, are usually estrogen dependent, often difficult to diagnose on a mammogram, and have a slightly higher risk of being in both breasts.

Newer classification schemes

Recently it has become clear that a classification according to how cells look under the microscope does not give enough information about how the cancer will behave in the future. Cells have genes and molecular markers that act as the engines for the cell and determine how rapidly the cells will grow, whether they will spread, and in some cases how they will respond to treatment. Molecular classifications of tumours provide more information and may allow the oncologist to make more individualized treatment recommendations. Using both molecular and pathological features provides a better ability to predict a cancer's future behaviour.

The current important molecular, pathological, and clinical features to consider are:
- Hormone receptors: positive or negative
- HER2 overexpression: present or absent

- Tumour grade: Grade 1, 2, 3 (low, moderate, or high). Markers such as Ki67 or MIB1 may be reported and usually give another indication of grade
- Extent of disease: limited or more extensive (see Chapter 16)
- Other features

Hormone receptors

Breast cancers are tested to see if they are sensitive to hormones. Approximately 75% of breast cancers have hormone receptors. Cancers that have hormone receptors respond to the female hormones, estrogen and progesterone. When stimulated with these hormones the tumour cells grow and divide. Estrogen receptors are the most common receptors and predict whether the tumour will respond to anti-estrogen therapy (see Chapter 27). Progesterone receptors are less common and seem to work with the estrogen receptor to make the cell more responsive to hormonal treatment. Hormone receptors may be reported as 1+, 2+ or 3+ or by a system known as the Allred score that gives a number from 0 to 8. An Allred estrogen receptor score of 7 to 8 out of 8 is the same as a 3+ score. An Allred score of less than 3 out of 8 is considered negative.

HER2 overexpression

HER2 is a cancer gene. In 15 to 20% of breast cancers this gene is overexpressed, which means that there is too much HER2 in the cell. Studies have shown that breast cancers with HER2 overexpression behave in a more aggressive manner, growing more quickly and often travelling to other sites of the body. As well, studies have suggested that HER2 over-expressing cancers may respond differently to some of our standard cancer treatments. A drug that specifically targets HER2 (trastuzumab or Herceptin, see Chapter 39) is used to reduce the chance of cancer recurring after surgery or to treat patients in whom the cancer has recurred. There are a number of other anti-HER2 drugs being developed, but the only one other than Herceptin that is licensed is lapatinib (Tykerb), which is approved for recurrent HER2-positive breast cancer (see Chapter 28).

Grade

When the pathologist examines the cancer under a microscope, a number of features are assessed which together help us predict how quickly the cancer will grow. Considering these features, the pathologist may use a grading system that gives the cancer a score. Some pathologists report grade on a scale of one to three and others on a scale of three to nine. Cancers may be low grade (score 1 out of 3, or 3 to 5 out of 9), moderate grade (score 2 out of 3, or 6 to 7 out of 9) or high grade (score 3 out of 3, or 8 to 9 out of 9). "Low grade" refers to a slower growing cancer. "Moderate" describes a medium growing cancer, while a cancer that appears very abnormal and is likely to grow quickly is classified as "high grade." Newer methods of assessing grade include staining the cancer for other "genetic" markers such as Ki67. Some doctors recommend that a Ki67 of greater than 13% be considered a higher risk cancer (similar to Grade 3). But this is not standard and there is no agreement about the cutoff level to define a fast growing cancer from a less aggressive cancer.

Extent of disease at diagnosis: Limited versus more extensive

A number of features are used to determine the extent of the disease, including:
- Size: The larger the cancer, the more likely it is to spread. Breast cancers are classified as "small" when they are up to 2 cm in diameter, "medium" if they are between 2 and 5 cm and "large" if they are bigger than 5 cm. If the cancer is invading into the skin or growing into the muscle or chest wall it is called "locally advanced" and has a higher risk of recurring or spreading.
- Nodes: Cancer cells can travel and the first place they may spread is into the lymph nodes. The risk of the cancer spreading to other parts of the body is related to the number of armpit (axillary) lymph nodes that are found to have cancer. The risk of spread is also related to the amount of cancer in the lymph nodes. The risk is higher if there are multiple, large lymph nodes filled with cancer compared, for example, to a millimetre of cancer in one node. The cancer may also extend from the lymph node into the fat in the armpit, which may increase the risk of the cancer recurring in the armpit.
- Lymphatic or vascular invasion: If cancer cells are found in the lymph channels or blood vessels in the breast, the prognosis is similar to having one involved lymph node in the axilla.

Other features

To more effectively predict how a cancer is going to behave, many researchers assess other features that can contribute extra information. These include a number of ways of assessing how quickly the cell is growing such as "mitotic index," percent of cells in "S-phase" and "ploidy." Other molecular features such as the presence of the genes p53 or p27 may be determined. In addition, some laboratories and companies are starting to look at a technique called *microarray analysis*, which assesses a large number of genes that the breast cancer may "over" or "under" express. This means that a cancer may have too much or too little of a gene and this may affect how it grows. These tests may prove to be very important in the next few years but at this time are not used on an everyday basis. Two genetic expression-based tests that are being tested for their ability to predict the risk of the cancer coming back and select appropriate treatment are the Oncotype Recurrence Score and the Mammoprint test (see Chapter 30).

Rare Types of Invasive Cancer

Inflammatory cancer

Inflammatory cancer is an aggressive form of cancer that presents with a red or swollen breast that may look like an infection. Inflammatory breast cancer cells spread rapidly through the lymph channels in the breast and skin causing the breast to become swollen, enlarged, and tender and the skin to get warm and red. Any woman who appears to have a breast infection (unless she is breast-feeding and has mastitis) should be checked promptly to exclude the possibility of inflammatory cancer. A mammogram may show thickening of the skin, but the diagnosis is made with a biopsy.

Sarcomas

Sarcomas are tumours that come from connective tissue such as nerves, fat, fibrous tissue, or blood vessels of the breast rather than the milk ducts. Cystosarcoma phylloides may be benign or malignant depending on the number of cells that are seen dividing when the tumour is examined under the microscope. This tumour is usually cured by surgery with either a partial or full mastectomy depending on the size of the tumour and its location. It is important that the tumour is completely removed as these tumours can cause problems by regrowing in the original site or on the chest wall.

PART TWO | **What are my options now that I have a diagnosis of breast cancer?**

An overview of treatment

CHAPTER FIFTEEN

An overview of breast cancer treatment

Is there more than one way to treat breast cancer?

YOU MAY FEEL CONFUSED TO LEARN that the treatment recommended to you for breast cancer is different from what others have received. For example, your aunt may have had a mastectomy, while a friend was treated with chemotherapy and radiation first, followed by mastectomy while another friend might have had a lumpectomy, radiation, and tamoxifen.

Why all these different approaches? What do these different treatments mean? What is the best treatment for you?

When a breast cancer is diagnosed there are three major decisions to be made:

1. What to do regarding your breast: save it (breast conserving surgery) or remove it (mastectomy).
2. What to do regarding the lymph nodes in your armpit (nothing, surgery, radiation, or both surgery and radiation).
3. What to do regarding treatment of the rest of the body (nothing, chemotherapy, hormone therapy, Herceptin, or a combination of chemotherapy, hormone therapy, and Herceptin).

The best decisions about these three issues will depend on the type and extent (or stage) of cancer, your ability to tolerate the treatments, and your preferences.

If the cancer is confined to the breast and lymph nodes in the armpit, the primary therapy is usually surgery (see Chapter 19) aimed at removing the cancerous tissues. Sometimes, however, pre-operative chemotherapy, also called *neoadjuvant*, is recommended (see Chapter 29), especially in cases where the tumour is large or it is known that the lymph nodes are involved. The important decision about the type of surgery to be used, either mastectomy or an approach that saves the breast, requires your input (see Chapter 20).

Once the cancer has been removed, an estimate of the prognosis of the cancer can be determined from the pathologist's examination of the cancerous tissue (see Chapters 12 to 14). A recommendation for additional treatment, called *adjuvant therapy* (see Chapter 22) is based on weighing the likelihood that your cancer will grow back after the surgery against the chance of unnecessary side effects caused by too much treatment.

If the risk of regrowth in the local area (breast or chest wall and lymph nodes) is substantial, then adjuvant radiation therapy is used (see Chapters 24 and 25). To reduce the chance of recurrence elsewhere in the body, additional treatment with drugs (hormones, chemotherapy, or Herceptin; see Chapters 27 and 30) is offered, except to those women with the very lowest risk of recurrence. If recurrence in both the local area and throughout the rest of the body is a concern, combined adjuvant therapy may be recommended—for example, radiation to the breast after a lumpectomy plus chemotherapy, with or without Herceptin, or hormonal therapy.

CHAPTER SIXTEEN

Staging and prognosis

What is staging?

AFTER THE DIAGNOSIS OF CANCER has been made it is important to determine the extent or stage of the cancer before deciding on the treatment plan. Briefly, a cancer that is small and confined to the breast is at an early stage, and one that has spread to other parts of the body is advanced or metastatic. Based on knowledge of the extent of the disease, your surgeon or oncologist (cancer specialist) can make recommendations about the chances of being cured by surgery alone, the type of surgery that is likely to give you the best possible outcome, and whether additional treatments (radiation, hormones, chemotherapy, or Herceptin) will be helpful.

The physical examination

Staging starts with a physical examination by your doctor. Your lungs, liver, abdomen, back, and limbs will be examined for abnormalities. Your breast will be examined and any lumps will be measured. Your armpit and neck will be felt to see if any lymph nodes are enlarged. Not all enlarged lymph nodes are cancerous: the doctor will try to determine this by assessing whether a node feels normal or enlarged, soft or hard, and whether it is movable. If a suspicious lymph node is found, a fine-needle aspiration may be done (see Chapter 10). Unfortunately, simple physical examination is not foolproof, and sometimes cancerous lymph nodes are not found until surgery.

Blood tests

Blood tests will be done to check whether your bone marrow, liver, and kidneys are working normally. Some doctors also order blood tests to look for tumour markers, which are proteins that leak out of cancer cells and can be measured in the blood. These markers are not reliable for diagnosing cancer, but occasionally suggest metastases. The markers that may be measured in breast cancer are CA15.3 (cancer antigen 15.3), CEA (carcinoembryonic antigen), and CA125.

Other tests

A chest X-ray should be taken to check the condition of the lungs and to check for any benign or malignant lung disease. For older women, an electrocardiogram (ECG) may be done to check the heart before surgery or chemotherapy.

A bone scan is only necessary for women who have a high risk of metastasis to the bones, or who have symptoms of spread to the bones (such as a new localized pain). The same goes for ultrasound or CT examinations of the liver. A liver ultrasound is not done routinely. PET scans are not routinely recommended but may be used for staging of patients with very high risk breast cancer where there is a suspicion of cancer spread beyond the breast. Some breast cancers, however, do not light up with a PET scan, and even a PET scan cannot show very small amounts of cancer in the lymph nodes. There is no test at this time that can prove that individual cancer cells have not spread out of the breast.

Official systems of staging

There are several systems for classifying the extent or stage of breast cancer. The two most common are the Stage I, II, III, IV system (Table 5) and the TNM system (Table 6).

It is important to recognize that staging systems only provide estimates of the chances for survival. The numbers are just averages. They can not be used to determine the exact outcome for a particular woman. Each case is unique and other details of your own case, not just the size and location of the tumour, are used

Table 5 **Historical stage definitions (I to IV) of breast cancer**	
Definition	**Average 5-year survival with treatment**
Stage I Tumour 2 cm or less, no metastases, no cancer in lymph nodes	80 to 95%
Stage II Tumour 2 to 5 cm but not involving skin and chest wall. If lymph nodes are involved they must be movable	50 to 70%
Stage III Advanced local tumour, fixed to the skin or chest wall, or presence of lymph nodes "attached" to structures in the axilla or enlarged above the collarbone	30 to 60%
Stage IV Cancer spread beyond the breast and axilla, to distant organs	5 to 20%

to help determine the chance of being cured by surgery alone or with additional therapy. As well, the different subtypes of breast cancer (whether they are estrogen sensitive or HER2 overexpressing) also affect outcome regardless of stage. In other words, these staging systems, although important, are most useful to describe the extent of disease at the time of diagnosis and to help plan the treatment strategy.

The Stage I, II, III, IV system

This simple system defines four stages of breast cancer (see Table 5). Stage I represents early cancer, with a small tumour and no spread to the lymph nodes in the armpit. In stages II and III, the tumour is progressively more advanced, while stage IV refers to metastatic disease that has spread to other areas of the body.

Since each stage (I to IV) is rather broad, the survival expectation within each stage is quite variable. For example, for a woman with stage I cancer, the average survival at 5 years after diagnosis is 85%. However, within this category there could be a woman with a mammographically detected cancer of just 0.5 cm in diameter as well as another woman with a 2 cm diameter, Grade 3 cancer invading the lymphatic vessels in the breast. The first woman would have a 95% chance of living free of cancer for over 10 years while the second woman would have a survival expectation closer to that of women with stage II tumours (a 30 to 50% chance of recurrence within five years).

A note of caution: the *grade* (on a scale of 1 to 3) of the tumour refers to the appearance of the cancer cells under the microscope and should not be confused with the *stage* or extent of the cancer (on a scale of I to IV).

Table 6   The TNM staging system

Tumour Stages: (T)

T(0):	no identifiable tumour in the breast
Tis:	in situ (non-invasive) cancer only
T(1a):	invasive cancer 5 mm or less in diameter
T(1b):	invasive cancer 6 to 10 mm in diameter
T(1c):	invasive cancer 11 to 20 mm in diameter
T(2):	invasive cancer 2 to 5 cm in diameter
T(3):	invasive cancer larger than 5 cm without skin or chest wall involvement
T(4a):	tumour of any size fixed to the chest wall
T(4b):	tumour of any size invading the skin
T(4c):	tumour of any size invading both chest wall and the skin
T(4d):	inflammatory cancer

Node Stages: (N)

N(0):	no evidence of palpable lymph nodes
N(1):	palpable, mobile lymph nodes in the armpit only or 1 to 3 nodes positive at axillary sampling
N(2):	lymph nodes in the axilla are fixed to each other or to adjacent structures such as nerves, muscles, skin, or bones, or 4 to 9 lymph nodes positive at axillary sampling
N(3):	involved lymph nodes beside the breast bone or above the collarbone or more than 9 lymph nodes positive at axillary dissection

Metastasis Stages: (M)

M(0):	no evidence of metastases
M(1):	metastases are present

The TNM system

The TNM system defines the extent of the cancer at the time of diagnosis based on three features of the tumour: the size/extent of the primary tumour (T), the extent of lymph node involvement (N), and the presence or absence of metastases (M). There are nine possible T categories, four N categories, and two M categories. This system is not as simple as the stage I, II, III, IV system for everyday use, but it is useful for cancer specialists to communicate with each other.

CHAPTER SEVENTEEN

Strategies for navigating the cancer care system

THE TREATMENT OF BREAST CANCER involves many different health care providers. Most patients assume these people work as part of a well-coordinated team but, unfortunately, this is not often the case. Each professional is qualified in her or his field, but they often work in relative isolation.

Find a helper if you can

In most situations, there is no single medical person who functions in the role of "case manager" to coordinate a patient's medical files and her passage through the treatment system. Many patients assume that their general practitioner (GP) will take on this role, but it is not a responsibility that many GPs can assume. Not all medical reports are automatically forwarded to the GP and, of those that are, some may be slow in arriving. In addition, even though breast cancer is the most common form of cancer in women, each GP may have only one or two patients with a new diagnosis of breast cancer each year. The GP may not feel well equipped to handle the details of the multiple options facing a woman with breast cancer. As a result, many patients find that they need someone, other than themselves, to act as a case manager to help them sift, organize, integrate, and keep track of all the information, advice, and appointments they encounter.

Some suggest that the patient herself would make the best case manager since she knows the most about her history and any special health problems. However, most cancer treatments subject the patient to a high degree of physical and psychological strain. Thus, the addition of case-management responsibilities to this load creates a huge additional burden. If possible, it is best to have a second person involved.

Typically, the person who takes on this role is a spouse, partner, relative, or close friend. No medical background is necessary, although it helps. The most important thing is a willingness to devote the time and attention needed to help the patient.

To be most helpful, the case manager needs to accompany the patient to most, if not all, appointments, tests and procedures. Almost all health care providers will allow the case manager to stay with the patient if the patient asks. See "Helpful hints for the case manager" below.

Questions to ask about surgery

When a breast cancer is diagnosed the first treatment is usually surgery. It is important to ask questions regarding surgery and to take time to make your decision.
1. Why is this surgery being recommended? Are there other options? What is the risk of the cancer returning with this surgery? Will I need other treatment like radiation therapy?
2. Should I be considering a mastectomy and reconstruction? A mastectomy? A lumpectomy?
3. How long will I be in hospital? What is my recovery going to involve?
4. When will I see a radiation oncologist? Medical oncologist?

Questions to ask about drug treatments, radiation, and other therapy

When the patient has been prescribed a new drug or treatment as part of her breast cancer care, the case manager should ask specific questions of the physician, pharmacist, or nurse before the patient begins taking the drug. These questions should also be asked of any alternative health care practitioner the patient may be seeing, such as a naturopath who has prescribed alternative therapies, e.g., herbal remedies or vitamins.

1. Why is this drug or treatment being prescribed?
2. What is the goal of the therapy? Is it for cure? Is it to slow disease? Is it to relieve symptoms?
3. Is this a standard or a new therapy? What is the evidence for using this particular protocol?
4. How and when do we know if the treatment is working? How long should it be continued?
5. What happens if the treatment doesn't work? Should it be stopped or the dose increased?
6. Are there other treatment options?
7. What are the potential harmful effects? How should we recognize and manage them?
8. Who should we call if there are problems or if we have more questions?

A word about the Internet

The Internet is a mixed blessing because it contains almost as much potentially harmful information as it does helpful information. Your specialist or the librarian at your local cancer treatment centre may be able to direct you to websites that provide credible information.

Helpful hints for the case manager

Some duties that a case manager could undertake with the patient's consent:

- Take a notebook and recording device to all appointments. (Ask for permission from the doctor or care provider before recording.)
- Keep a written record of all the instructions to the patient.
- Keep a record of all the tests that are ordered and of all appointments. This may avoid duplication of testing.
- Ask for copies of all the medical and pathology reports. This is the patient's right under the freedom of information laws in most places. Keep them all in a binder. Understand these are used to record results and may not include instructions.
- Speak up when you are becoming frustrated with information overload or conflicting information. If necessary, put your concerns in writing (tactfully and positively).

- Carry a cell phone if you can't be easily reached.
- Remember that the patient's medical files are not routinely passed from one health care facility to another unless the patient or physician requests specific information. Ensure that the patient informs the health care provider of any special problems or conditions that have arisen since the last visit, including new medications, allergy alerts, or reactions to tests or anaesthetics.
- If possible, secure other sources of information and support from health care providers who are not directly involved with the patient's care. These people can be valuable sources of medical knowledge and insight.
- Encourage the patient to have a good relationship with her family physician. Although the specialist will direct most of the cancer specific treatments, it is the family physician who maintains contact with the patient when her cancer treatments are completed. As well, the family physician should receive results of tests and can be called to get results prior to the next appointment with the oncologist.
- Before the patient sees a specialist such as a surgeon or oncologist, fax or email any questions you have. Because of their busy schedules, they may find it helpful to receive the questions in writing and in advance of the appointment.
- The patient may want to invest in "call display" so she can answer only the calls that she chooses, while leaving the others for you to respond to when time allows.
- Your responsibility is not to become a medical expert but an expert on what has happened (treatments, patient moods, test results, etc.) in relation to the patient.
- Maintain a calm, caring presence for the sake of the patient and yourself.
- Almost every health care provider is a skilled expert, but is probably overworked with more than the optimal number of patients. They are doing their best and your goal is to help them achieve this. Positive comments expressing your appreciation are most helpful.
- Allow friends and relatives to help you and give you support. It is essential that you do not "burn out" so consider your own needs and take good care of yourself.

The surgical options

Chapter Eighteen

The doctor has suggested surgery:
What should I do?

TODAY'S OPERATIONS ARE MUCH LESS EXTENSIVE than in the past. When it comes to surgery, more is not necessarily better. There is usually a team of experts who treat the cancer with a combination of surgery, radiation, chemotherapy, hormones, and Herceptin. You are also part of the team and have a role to play—learning about the disease, hearing the options, discussing your needs with your family and friends, and coming to a comfortable decision about what you want.

After finding a lump, long delays to start treatment are not advised, but you should not be rushed or pushed into accepting a treatment plan before you are ready, even if it means waiting an extra week or so for surgery to obtain a second opinion or to make up your mind about treatment options. It is best to feel well informed and confident.

Why surgery?

Surgical removal of the breast cancer is an important cornerstone in the treatment of breast cancer. Some women may be completely cured by surgery alone. However, removal of the tumour, combined with radiation therapy, often provides better control of the cancer than with either surgery or radiation therapy used alone. In addition, examination of the tissues removed during surgery provides important information about the type and size of the cancer, the extent of lymph node involvement and the level of estrogen receptors. This information allows the oncologist to determine the stage of the cancer and to tailor any further treatment to your particular case.

For some cancers, surgery is not the best initial treatment. If the tumour is locally advanced, meaning that there is either a very large breast lump or very enlarged lymph nodes, or it is the inflammatory type of cancer, chemotherapy and radiation may be given first to reduce the size of the tumour. Afterward, mastectomy may be recommended to further reduce the risk of cancer recurrence in the breast. Chemotherapy may also be given prior to surgery (called *neoadjuvant* chemotherapy) in situations where it is clear that chemotherapy will be recommended.

In the uncommon situation when the cancer has already spread (metastasized) beyond both the breast and lymph node areas, the initial treatment may include hormones, chemotherapy, radiation, or Herceptin, or a combination of some or all of these treatments, rather than surgery.

Choosing a surgeon

How can you find the best surgeon for you? Usually, one surgeon cannot be singled out who is best for everyone in all circumstances. The ideal surgeon is knowledgeable about breast surgery and current practices as well as being skillful in the operating room. Your surgeon should be someone with whom you feel confident.

Many patients are referred to their surgeon through their family doctor. This is fine provided you have confidence in both your family physician and his or her choice. In almost every sizable community there are surgeons who have a special interest in breast cancer. Good information about surgeons can be obtained from women volunteering with the Breast Cancer Visitors program of the Cancer Society or other local support and advocacy groups for breast cancer. You should be able to ask the surgeon questions and get satisfactory answers. If you are not comfortable, however, do not be afraid to request a second opinion.

Many cancer centres have breast cancer policy groups. Surgeons participating in such a group will be aware of current trends and practices and may be better able to respond to your questions.

CHAPTER NINETEEN

Types of breast surgery

THERE ARE MANY TYPES OF SURGERY AVAILABLE for the treatment of breast cancer. Each procedure has its advantages and disadvantages, depending on the situation. The type of operation best for you depends on a combination of factors: the type of cancer, its size and location, your preference, the surgeon's preference, and the policies of the hospital or cancer centre where the treatment takes place.

Take time to consider your options

While it is true that you shouldn't delay surgery too long, most cancers have been present for a number of years and there is no need to rush into the operating room by nightfall. A delay of one to two weeks is usually less important than careful consideration of the surgical options. You should understand your choices and feel comfortable with them. There is time for a well thought out choice based on careful examination of the options, discussions with other patients, a second opinion if desired, and an evaluation of your needs with your family and friends.

It is unwise to assume that you can't understand the details of the treatment and give up control because of feelings of anxiety or fear. Spend a few days talking with others and thinking about which route is best for you. Taking this time to decide what you want leads to an informed choice that ensures that you remain confident and have some measure of control. In the long run, this is time well spent.

Breast Surgery

Breast surgery includes operations on the breast and operations on the lymph nodes under the armpit. Operations on the breast remove the breast cancer and allow examination of the cancer as well as the surrounding tissue. Another important part of breast surgery is a procedure to assess whether cancer has spread into the lymph nodes under the armpit. If the cancer has spread into the lymph nodes, the diseased lymph nodes are generally removed.

Operations that save the breast (breast-conserving surgery)

Partial mastectomy: removing a small amount of the breast

A partial mastectomy (also known as *lumpectomy*, *segmental mastectomy*, or *wide excision*) is an operation that removes the cancer plus some surrounding normal breast tissue (Figure 18). This has become the most commonly performed surgery for the treatment of early breast cancer. Studies have found that a partial mastectomy that removes the entire cancer followed by radiation gives a woman the same chance of survival and control of the cancer as does an operation that removes the whole breast.

When the cancer and breast tissue are taken out, careful attention is paid to the edges (margins) of the tissue being removed to make certain that they don't contain any cancer. The objective is to remove the cancer lump along with any of the "tentacles" that extend into the normal breast tissue while still leaving enough tissue so that the breast looks cosmetically normal.

After a skillfully done partial mastectomy for a small tumour, the breast should look similar to the untreated breast (Figure 19). The size of the area removed depends partly on the location of the tumour and the size of the breast. The goal of the surgery is to remove the cancer but leave the breast as normal-appearing as possible. Ask your surgeon how much normal tissue will be removed. In general, removal of more than 1.0 to 1.5 cm of tissue beyond the cancer itself is rarely required. However, it is not always possible

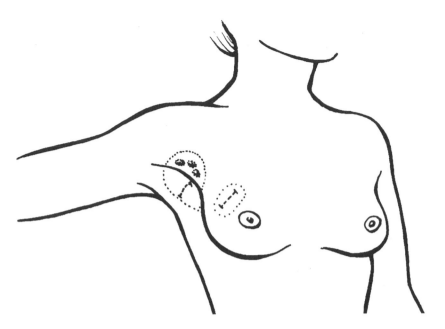

Figure 18: A partial mastectomy involves removing some normal breast tissue surrounding the cancer. The axillary dissection is performed through a separate incision in the armpit.

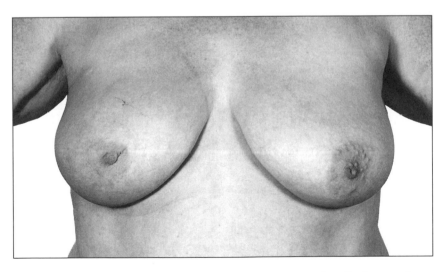

Figure 19: Five years after a partial mastectomy and radiotherapy for a cancer of the right breast.

to know the exact extent of the cancer in the breast before the operation. If the edges of the lumpectomy contain tumour cells, more surgery, either a re-excision of the breast tissue, or a mastectomy may be recommended. Removal of an excessive amount of normal tissue will adversely affect the way your breast will look after surgery.

Operations that remove the breast

Total mastectomy

A total mastectomy is the removal of the entire breast and nipple. No muscle is removed. This procedure is used when there is evidence that the cancer is too large to remove with a partial mastectomy or when the patient chooses to have the whole breast removed as a personal preference. A total mastectomy may also be performed for a woman who has a strong family history of breast cancer and decides to have both breasts removed to eliminate the risk of developing breast cancer (not a decision to be taken lightly). A *simple mastectomy* often has the same meaning as a *total mastectomy* but it is an antiquated term that could suggest that less breast tissue would be removed.

During a total mastectomy, an incision is made over the breast. The resulting scar, after removal of the breast and lymph nodes, is long and straight or diagonal across the chest wall (Figure 20). Ask your surgeon how the scar will look and what measures he or she can take to make it easier for you to consider reconstructive surgery if you decide to have it later. A total mastectomy is usually done under general anaesthetic and often requires a night in hospital. The armpit lymph nodes are removed and a drain tube is left in place to avoid fluid build-up.

Subcutaneous, skin-sparing, and nipple-sparing mastectomies

These mastectomies have been used to prevent future cancer risk in women who are at high risk for the development of breast cancer, and are usually performed in conjunction with breast reconstruction under one general anaesthetic. In the subcutaneous mastectomy, the tissue is removed through a small incision while preserving the skin and the nipple of the breast. The main disadvantage of this operation is that there will be some breast tissue left behind the nipple and sometimes at the edges of the breast. There

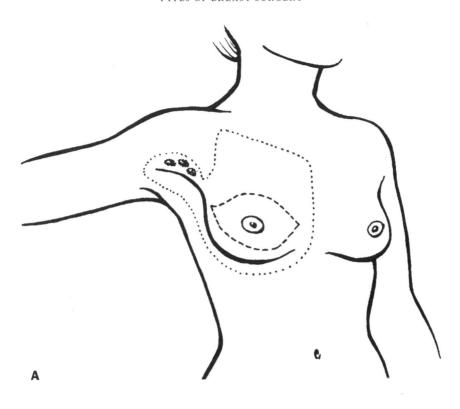

A

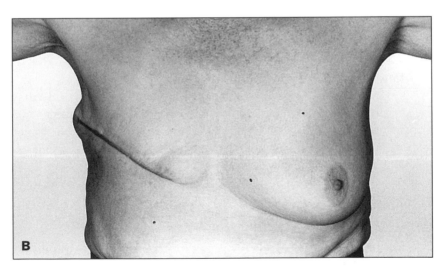

B

Figure 20: Extent of tissue removed (A) and appearance after a total mastectomy (B).

is concern that cancer could develop in that remaining tissue. A variant of the subcutaneous mastectomy is the nipple-sparing mastectomy, in which there is a plan to remove all the breast tissue but leave the skin and nipple with less breast tissue behind the nipple. This type of surgery usually includes a biopsy of the tissue just underneath the nipple to ensure that no disease has spread along the milk ducts into the remaining residual nipple. A disadvantage of the nipple-sparing surgery is that the nerves to the nipple are cut and the nipple does not have any feeling afterwards. In addition, unless the patient is young with excellent breast shape prior to surgery, the spared nipple may not end up in an optimum location.

The skin-sparing mastectomy is a variant of the total mastectomy in which the nipple is removed but the breast skin is preserved. This "envelope" is usually filled with some tissue or an implant to provide an immediate form of reconstruction.

Radical mastectomy

A radical mastectomy is an old treatment that was popular more than 50 years ago. It included removal of the breast, muscles underneath the breast, some nerves, the nipple, the skin, and all the lymph nodes in the armpit right up to the collar bone. Sometimes a skin graft was needed because so much tissue was removed. The chance of swelling due to fluid retention, called lymphedema, was high. These days a radical mastectomy is very rarely necessary.

Mastectomy and immediate reconstruction

Many women who need or desire a mastectomy (see Chapter 20) may also be interested in reconstruction (see Chapter 34). It may be possible to perform the reconstruction at the same time as the mastectomy (called *immediate reconstruction*). The potential for reconstruction or immediate reconstruction should be discussed prior to mastectomy.

Removal and assessment of lymph nodes in the armpit: Sentinel lymph node biopsy and axillary dissection

Along with removal of the tumour from the breast, lymph nodes are usually removed from the armpit. There are two reasons for determining whether any disease has spread to the lymph nodes. First, if cancer has spread to the lymph nodes, it influences the need for and type of chemotherapy, radiation therapy, or hormone therapy that is offered after surgery. Second, removal of any diseased lymph nodes improves disease control for the region. Lymph nodes that contain disease may continue to grow in spite of other treatments and cause severe problems in the future. If left untreated, diseased lymph nodes can obstruct the blood vessels and damage the nerves to the hand and arm and also cause swelling of the arm and breast. Thankfully this problem can usually be avoided if the diseased nodes are surgically removed. If there are many nodes with disease, radiation can also be added to further reduce recurrence.

There are generally two procedures involved with the assessment and surgical treatment of the axilla: sentinel node biopsy and axillary dissection. Over the last few years, sentinel lymph node biopsy has become accepted as the standard technique to assess whether cancer cells have spread to the lymph nodes under the arm. Sentinel lymph node biopsy involves the mapping and labeling of axillary lymph nodes with a radioactive tracer or blue dye (or both) that is injected into the breast around the nipple area or around the cancer. These two dyes are absorbed into the lymphatic channels of the breast and travel to the first few lymph nodes under the armpit and are trapped there. The position of these sentinel lymph nodes is determined using a special electronic probe in the operating room. A small incision is made over the labeled nodes and one to five sentinel nodes are removed and examined under the microscope to see if there is any involvement with cancer.

Since 2000, surgeons who have specialized in breast cancer surgery have learned and improved the methodology for sentinel node biopsy. Breast surgical oncologists have considerable expertise in this technique. There is close integration between the surgeon, nuclear medicine department, and pathologist. Studies have shown that there is a relatively small chance that cancer cells will be missed using this technique. No method is without some chance of error but sentinel node biopsy is considered accurate and associated with many fewer arm problems than a full dissection of all of the lymph nodes under the armpit. Sentinel node biopsy is most useful for solitary breast cancers less than 5 cm in diameter when there are no suspicious or positive lymph nodes felt in the armpit. If the cancer is large or invading the skin or muscles or if the surgeon can feel enlarged or suspicious nodes in the axilla, a sentinel node biopsy may not be accurate. If lymph nodes feel suspicious prior to surgery then they are probably best assessed by a fine needle or core biopsy using palpation or ultrasound as a guide.

If there is disease in the sentinel node, the standard procedure has been to remove 6 to 15 additional lymph nodes from under the arm with an axillary dissection. About 20 to 30% of patients with a positive sentinel node will have other lymph nodes with disease in the axilla. Removal or treatment of the diseased lymph nodes is considered important for breast cancer control. The number of lymph nodes with disease is still the most important prognostic factor in determining the type of chemotherapy, radiation therapy, or hormone therapy that is offered. In 2011, a large surgical study found that women who had no further surgery after being found to have one or two positive sentinel nodes had similar cancer control and survival compared to women who had a completion axillary dissection. This study is leading to changes in the recommendations about the need for axillary dissection.

The axilla is divided into three levels. Usually the first two levels of lymph nodes are removed in an axillary node dissection. A properly performed axillary dissection usually contains more than ten lymph nodes, although this number is variable and often can depend on how carefully the pathologist looks for the small nodes. The deepest lymph nodes, found just below the collar bone (the level three nodes) are usually not removed unless they are grossly diseased. An axillary dissection is usually done under general anaesthetic and may require a night or more in the hospital. A separate incision is made in the armpit that is longer than for a sentinel lymph node biopsy (Figure 18). Just before closing the wound the surgeon places a small tube, or drain, into the area from which the lymph nodes were removed. The drainage tube is to collect fluid that would otherwise accumulate. The other end of the tube comes out through the skin and is sewn in place. The patient is usually discharged from hospital with this drain in place and given instructions on drain care. Usually community or home-care nurses are provided to help with drain management and wound care. After a few days, when less fluid is draining though the tube, the drain is removed.

CHAPTER TWENTY

What type of surgery is best for me?

Does one type of surgery offer a better chance of cure?

THE AIM OF SURGERY is to give you the best chance of being cured of cancer. Usually, the choice is between breast conservation (a partial mastectomy) or breast removal (called *total* or *modified-radical mastectomy*) as described in Chapter 19. Studies have shown that partial mastectomy followed by radiation therapy and a total mastectomy provide an equal chance of cure and a high chance (90 to 95%) of controlling the cancer in the breast or chest wall. Therefore, your choice of operation need *not* be based on the relapse rate or chance of having the cancer come back. With either option a sentinel node biopsy or an axillary dissection if there is disease in the axillary (armpit) lymph nodes is standard.

How do I choose the right surgery?

A partial mastectomy is suitable for 75 to 85% of patients. Usually a woman will feel better about herself if she can keep her breast, but there are a number of other factors you and your surgeon should consider:
- Your preference
- The surgical issues, including the size of the breast, size of the tumour, its location, and the type of cancer cells

- Your age and general health
- Your ability to undergo radiation

Your preference counts

Whenever possible, *your preference* should be the deciding factor. A total mastectomy may seem like the better solution for a woman whose breasts are difficult to examine or who is "never going to trust that breast again." On the other hand, a partial mastectomy conserves the breast and avoids the discomfort and necessity of wearing an artificial breast (prosthesis). The main disadvantages of a partial mastectomy are the inconvenience and side effects of several weeks of daily radiation treatments that are usually required after a breast-saving operation (see Chapters 24 to 26). Studies have shown that when women are fully informed of the risks and benefits of breast conservation and mastectomy and are given a choice, about 85% elect to save the breast.

Studies have also shown that in the years after surgery, women have similar levels of distress regardless of whether they have had their breast removed or saved. In other words, the diagnosis of cancer causes anxiety no matter what type of surgery is done. Other studies have shown that women who are given the choice of surgical treatment feel empowered and therefore adjust to the diagnosis of breast cancer more easily than women who are told to have a particular type of operation.

Surgical issues

Surgical considerations include the size and location of the tumour compared to the size of the breast. If the tumour is large and the breast is small, a partial mastectomy may remove too much breast tissue, leaving a disappointing cosmetic result. In general, tumours larger than 5 cm are better treated by a total mastectomy, with the option of breast reconstruction either later or at the same time. As a rule, tumours that are smaller than 3 cm can almost always be removed by a partial mastectomy. The size of the breast must be carefully considered for tumours between 3 and 5 cm. If the tumour is very large, it may be advisable to have chemotherapy and radiation before the surgery. If the tumour shrinks dramatically, it could still be possible to conserve the breast.

The location of the tumour can also affect the cosmetic result of a partial mastectomy. If the tumour is in the centre of the breast the nipple may have to be removed, resulting in a less satisfactory appearance as well as loss of nipple sensation. If the partial mastectomy is done well, however, the result may be superior to a mastectomy and reconstruction, or mastectomy and a prosthesis.

About 2 to 4% of women are found to have two or more tumours in one breast. If there are multiple tumours within the breast, it might not be possible to remove all the affected areas without removing the whole breast. Multiple tumours are usually identified before surgery on a mammogram or MRI, but sometimes they are only identified in the pathology report after surgery. If a mastectomy is felt to be the best choice and the tumour is not "locally advanced" it may be possible to do an immediate breast reconstruction during the same anaesthetic (see Chapter 34).

Your overall health affects your ability to undergo radiation

The state of your general health is an important factor when deciding if a partial mastectomy is the best treatment for you. Since radiation therapy is generally required after a partial mastectomy, breast conservation should not be recommended if you are not suitable for radiation. Radiation treatment may be difficult for someone who is elderly or very weak and has difficulty visiting a clinic every day for 3 to 6 weeks. Patients who cannot lie flat on the treatment table, or who cannot lift their arms over their head for the radiation treatment (for example after a stroke) will have difficulty with this part of the treatment. Therefore, they may be advised to have a total mastectomy instead.

You would also be considered unsuitable for radiation treatment if it were felt that you have a high risk of severe side effects (see Chapter 26). Some women who have certain medical conditions should generally not receive radiation therapy. These conditions include severe lung or heart disease, or systemic lupus erythematosus, scleroderma, or ataxia-telangiectasia. Women with the latter conditions may have severe reactions and scarring from the radiation and are often best treated by a total mastectomy. Women who are pregnant should avoid radiation therapy because of possible harm to the fetus and may be better treated with total mastectomy.

Women with very large breasts tend to get more radiation side effects because of the large amount of tissue that must be treated, but this must be weighed against the lopsided appearance that occurs if only one very large breast is removed with a mastectomy. Also, radiation should not be given to a woman who has already received therapeutic doses of radiation to the same breast in the past.

Partial mastectomy means regular follow-up visits

After a partial mastectomy and radiation, the breast should be carefully observed on a regular basis to detect any early, potentially curable cancer recurrence. You should get to know the normal feel of your treated breast. After surgery and radiation there are often areas of thickening or lumpiness. This is normal but you should report any *changes* in the lumpiness to your doctor. The best way to monitor your breasts is by regular breast self-examination. You should also have a physical examination every 6 to 12 months done by your family physician or a health care provider with experience in the follow-up of women after partial mastectomy and radiation.

A mammogram 6 months after the radiation treatment is completed may be recommended, followed by mammograms of both breasts annually. It is important that all women with breast cancer have regular mammograms unless both breasts have been removed.

Is a partial mastectomy better than a total mastectomy?

A breast-saving operation such as a partial mastectomy with sentinel lymph node biopsy (and axillary dissection if necessary) followed by radiation therapy to the breast provides an equal chance of cure and control of the disease as a total mastectomy with the same extent of axillary surgery. Six international scientific studies have confirmed this observation. This doesn't mean that a partial mastectomy is better, but it does allow you to make a choice. You should consider the risks and benefits of both, and your doctors should give you sufficient information and the respect to allow you to make an informed choice. Some authorities feel that breast conservation plus radiation therapy is preferable, since it achieves equal survival, and provides body image, sexual, and psychological advantages for the woman. Studies have shown that when offered a choice, about 85% of women elect to have a breast saving operation.

The advantage of a breast-saving operation is that the breast is saved. This must be weighed against the need for a series of radiation treatments that may require 3 to 6 weeks of daily visits to a cancer centre. The advantages of a total mastectomy are that the treatment is over at once and radiation treatments can be avoided in most cases. If there is a large cancer or more than one cancer in the affected breast, or if certain conditions make radiation more hazardous, total mastectomy may be the better option. A mastectomy means that the breast is removed completely. Since each person is unique, it is appropriate and healthy for you to participate in this crucial decision. But remember, if given the option, there is no "wrong" choice.

CHAPTER TWENTY-ONE

Hospitalization and recovering from surgery

Dealing with hospitalization

DEPENDING ON THE TYPE OF SURGERY YOU HAVE and your general health, you may be admitted to the hospital for the surgery only and sent home that day or stay for one or more nights. You may find the hospital's admission routine a source of frustration. Some patients feel that they are answering the same questions over and over again and wonder why nobody seems to be listening. Hospital procedures require that a patient be admitted by the clerk, the ward nurse, and a number of doctors, including the surgeon and anesthetist. In a teaching hospital the list may also include a student nurse, a medical student, an intern, and a resident. Be patient. They are listening, but each of them requires slightly different information. Also, the many questions ensure that everyone knows you individually and serves as a double or triple check that the correct procedure is planned, and that any allergies you suffer and medications that you take regularly are recorded.

The recovery room

In the recovery room nurses carefully monitor you as you wake up. Often, patients are confused for a short period. Also, you may have a sore throat. This is a temporary discomfort caused by the breathing tube that was used to help you breathe during the operation. The doctor will have provided a list of orders, including pain relief and other medications. You may feel nauseated from the anaesthetic or get shivers when you wake up. Don't hesitate to tell the nurses how you are feeling.

Your surgeon might come to talk to you here, although you may be too groggy to remember much. Only a few preliminary findings will be known right away. The full pathology report is usually not available for a few days. Some specialized tests on your tumour may take even longer.

Notifying your significant other

There is usually someone you will want the surgeon to contact when the operation is finished, so that person's name and phone number should be clearly written in your chart. If your significant other is waiting in the hospital, make sure it is clear exactly where they are since the surgeon may want to talk to them while you are in the recovery room.

The ward

The type of operation and your recovery time will determine how long you stay in hospital. Most patients go home the same day if the operation involved only the breast with or without a sentinel node biopsy. Even if a mastectomy and axillary dissection was needed, almost everyone will be able to go home the next morning. The sooner patients start moving around after surgery the fewer problems they have, so you will be urged to get out of bed and walk up and down the halls.

Nausea

Nausea is a common problem after breast surgery and a general anaesthetic. Tell your anesthesiologist and surgeon if you tend to develop severe nausea in these circumstances. There are new medications and techniques that may minimize this problem.

Pain

After the surgery there will be some pain that can be controlled with pain killers. Everyone is different, so let the nurse know when you are in pain so you can receive medication according to your needs. Many pain killers can cause nausea and constipation but this is generally mild and temporary.

Drains

If you have an axillary dissection or a mastectomy, you may have one or two drains in the area for the first few days to prevent fluid accumulation. The drains are usually checked and removed by a home care nurse several days after you leave hospital. Sometimes, after the drain is removed the fluid builds up again, causing a tender swelling in the armpit. This is called a *seroma*. The seroma may need to be drained using a syringe. This can be done easily in the clinic or surgeon's office during an outpatient visit.

Sutures

Some stitches (sutures) are designed to dissolve on their own while other non-absorbable sutures or staples need to be removed, usually a week to ten days after the surgery. Ask your surgeon what sort of sutures will be used. The redness of your scar will gradually fade over several months.

Going home: Ask questions before you leave

You are bound to have questions about what you can do when you get home, so write them down and be prepared to rattle off the list when you see your doctor after the surgery. Make sure you have a clear understanding about what you can and cannot do, what exercises you should do to start moving your arm, when to start them (see Chapter 33), when you should see the surgeon again, and when you will be referred to a medical or radiation oncologist. Also, be sure to have a prescription for pain killers because you may need them, especially as you get more active.

Most women suffer some pain along the incision and under the arm that lasts from several days to a few weeks or longer. This can be controlled with pain medications. Later on, some women experience a tightness or discomfort over the chest area which, although mild, is often bothersome and longer-lasting. This may be helped by physiotherapy (see Chapter 33). The incision usually heals within a few weeks, but can take somewhat longer in women who have had radiation before surgery.

The risk of infection with breast surgery is usually low, but if there is a foul-smelling drainage, increasingly red and tender skin, or any fever, there may be an infection and it should be treated promptly with antibiotics.

With any surgery, there is a risk of bleeding afterwards, even though the surgeon has been extremely careful. This can result in a hematoma (blood clot in the tissues), which can be swollen, painful, and leave the breast bruised-looking. Usually, the hematoma subsides on its own, but if it is large, it may need to be drained.

After breast surgery many women experience numbness in the back of the underarm or on the chest wall. This is usually due to nerves being cut or stretched during the operation and may improve in the months ahead.

Breast surgery is emotionally difficult for many women. Often, it is difficult for a patient to look at her own body, let alone show her spouse, friends, or family the scars. As the incision fades and you use your arm, you can begin to heal. A breast cancer support group and a physiotherapy consultation are often helpful to regain a positive sense of your body.

Visitors

A stay in hospital tends to bring friends and relatives out of the woodwork. Depending on your personality, this may or may not please you. If the visiting is too tiring, speak to your nurse and visitors can be restricted. Seeing people and discussing the situation can be helpful, especially with supportive people who are close to you, but do not let the socializing wear you out.

Obtaining a breast prosthesis

If you have been treated with a mastectomy, you may want to consider a prosthesis or breast reconstruction (see Chapter 34). The prosthesis is a soft, somewhat heavy plastic form that comes in many shapes and sizes to match the many shapes and sizes of women's breasts.

Breast Cancer Visitor volunteers from the Cancer Society will often supply a soft, fluffy breast form of cotton that you can wear temporarily in your own bra. This helps fill out your clothes but does not have the weight or shape of your other breast. A fitted prosthesis will help you feel better and walk straighter. Once the initial pain and swelling of the mastectomy has settled and the wound is healed, you are ready for a fitting. This is often 4 to 6 weeks after surgery.

Breast prostheses are not one-size-fits-all and just picking a form off the shelf will not give you the best fit. You need to consider the size, shape and weight of your remaining breast to get a good match. The traditional prosthesis is sold with a specially designed bra with a pocket into which the prosthesis can fit. A recent innovation is a prosthesis that directly adheres to the chest wall. It is attached to the chest by strips of Velcro that are glued to the chest and the underside of the prosthesis. Body heat activates the adhesive properties of the glue and the Velcro strips remain on the chest wall for a week to 10 days. They come off without the tearing or sting of usual adhesive plasters.

Additional garments are available such as bathing suits and nightgowns that are specially designed to hold the prosthesis.

Depending on where you live, there may be many or just a few places to buy a prosthesis such as department or drug stores. In larger towns you can find stores that specialize in selling and fitting prostheses and garments to wear with the prosthesis. Your surgeon, support group, local Cancer Society office, or nurses at your cancer centre should be able to direct you to a store. Breast prostheses are a medical appliance so you should check if the cost is covered by your medical insurance.

Preventing recurrence of cancer

Additional treatment following surgery: Radiation, chemotherapy, and hormone treatment

Why is additional treatment needed?

EVEN WHEN THE CANCER appears to have been totally removed, it is never possible to know that the surgeon "got it all." This is because microscopic cells may be in the remaining skin, breast tissue, or lymph nodes, or cancer cells may have got into the blood stream and spread elsewhere in the body as tiny, undetectable metastases. This is a frustrating problem because there is no known test that can detect a few residual cancer cells. Only time will tell whether the operation was indeed a cure.

Because of this uncertainty, treatment is given in addition to surgery as a preventive measure in case cancer cells are still present. This preventive treatment is called *adjuvant* therapy, and is a normal part of breast cancer treatment for the majority of women. Adjuvant therapy may be radiation, chemotherapy, Herceptin, hormonal agents, or various combinations of these treatments.

Who should receive adjuvant therapy?

Because we are not able to detect the presence of just a few microscopic cancer cells, each patient's risk of cancer recurrence is assessed based on the surgical findings and the pathology report (see Table 4, page 75).

Based on this assessment, adjuvant therapy may or may not be recommended to a particular patient. For instance, a woman with a very low risk of cancer recurrence and a high probability (more than 95%) of being cured by surgery alone may not require any adjuvant therapy. Adjuvant therapy recommendations are constantly being developed and refined to keep pace with the ever-improving understanding of breast cancer. However, most women today receive some form of adjuvant therapy.

When should adjuvant therapy start?

Adjuvant therapy is usually started within 4 to 12 weeks after surgery. It is sometimes difficult to accept the need for additional treatment so soon, especially because it requires one to admit the possibility of the cancer returning. Ideally, the concept of adjuvant therapy will have been discussed before surgery to give you more time to consider it and come to terms with the reasons for it.

Types of adjuvant therapy

Radiation therapy

Adjuvant radiation therapy is almost always given after partial mastectomy. Although the cancer may seem to have been removed completely, the likelihood of the cancer coming back in the same breast may be relatively high (10 to 40% over 10 years without radiation). Radiation to the breast can significantly reduce this risk.

Women who have had their breast removed may also be offered adjuvant radiation therapy if the tumour was large (more than 5 cm), if it was invading the skin or chest wall, or if lymph nodes removed from the axilla were cancerous. After mastectomy, adjuvant radiation decreases the chance of the cancer re-growing on the chest wall or in the lymph node areas, and may improve survival (see Chapter 25).

Chemotherapy

Chemotherapy is the use of drugs given orally, or more often, directly into a vein (see Chapters 29 to 31). Adjuvant chemotherapy is given after surgery if the risk of residual cancer cells in the body is relatively high due to the type or extent of the cancer, and the patient is fit enough to withstand the side effects, which vary with the type and dose of drugs used. Adjuvant chemotherapy decreases the risk of recurrence and increases the number of women who may be cured.

Hormone therapy

Hormone therapy is usually given as pills and can be effective against breast cancers that express either the estrogen or progesterone receptor, or both (see Chapter 12). Hormone therapy blocks estrogens from stimulating the growth of hormonally responsive cancer cells by either removing hormones from the body system or by making cancer cells less responsive to the actions of female hormones in the body. The connection between estrogen and cancer growth is discussed in Chapter 27. Hormone therapy is only effective if the tumour is sensitive to hormone stimulation (estrogen receptor or progesterone receptor positive) and may be used in either pre- or postmenopausal women. In premenopausal women, ovaries are the primary source of estrogen. Surgical removal of the ovaries or an injection to stop ovarian function may be recommended. After menopause the drug tamoxifen or the class of drugs called *aromotase inhibitors* may improve outcome.

Herceptin therapy

Herceptin (trastuzamab) adjuvant therapy is usually given as an intravenous injection every 3 weeks for a year or sometimes longer. Herceptin decreases the risk of recurrence and death for the 20 to 25% of women whose breast cancer overexpresses the HER2 gene. Herceptin has no benefit if the woman's tumour does not overexpress HER2. Other anti-HER2 drugs may also be used including in clinical trials.

Combined adjuvant therapy

Depending on the type of surgery and the type and extent of the breast cancer when it is discovered, more than one type of adjuvant therapy may be offered. Each woman's situation is different. Therefore, one woman may receive both radiotherapy and hormone therapy following her surgery, while another may get chemotherapy alone. When more than one type of adjuvant therapy is used, it is called *combined modality* treatment.

CHAPTER TWENTY-THREE

Treatment of in situ breast cancer

Treatment of ductal carcinoma in situ

BREAST CANCER THAT IS STILL ENTIRELY within the milk ducts of the breast and has not invaded nearby tissues is called *ductal carcinoma in situ* (DCIS). DCIS has not had a chance to spread to other parts of the body (see Chapter 13). DCIS is being diagnosed much more frequently today because of the increasing number of women having regular mammograms. In some individuals, DCIS might never progress to form an invasive cancer and might never be a threat to a woman's life. However, if left untreated, some cases of DCIS will become invasive and spread to other parts of the body.

The goal of treatment of DCIS is to completely remove or kill any cancer cells before they form an invasive cancer. If a breast-saving procedure is used, the aim of treatment is to have a less than 5% risk of recurrence in the breast during the first 10 years after surgery.

Breast conservation is an option

In the past, the traditional treatment for ductal carcinoma in situ was a total mastectomy to prevent the progression to invasive cancer. The cure rate after such a mastectomy is close to 100%. Mastectomy remains an acceptable treatment for DCIS. However, many women are interested in a treatment that conserves the breast and still provides an excellent chance for cure.

Studies have shown that radiation therapy to the breast after a partial mastectomy can significantly reduce the risk of cancer regrowing in the breast. For women who want to save their breast, partial mastectomy plus radiation is considered the standard treatment.

To remove the entire ductal carcinoma in situ but still save the breast, it is critical that the surgeon plan the operation with a clear idea of the mammogram appearance of the cancer. As well, the pathologist must systematically inspect many samples of the removed tissue to ensure that no invasive cancer is present and to give an estimate of whether the DCIS is likely to have been completely removed.

Radiation therapy has been shown to decrease the risk of regrowth of DCIS by about half. As a result, except in patients with the very lowest risk of recurrence, radiation therapy is usually recommended following a breast saving operation. Together, the surgery plus radiation provide a greater than 90% chance of local control of the cancer. If recurrence in the breast does develop, most cases may still be cured with a mastectomy.

The woman who chooses breast conservation requires lifelong follow-up so that if cancer does regrow in that breast, she can receive treatment at a stage when a cure is still possible. About half of the recurrences in the breast will be more DCIS and the rest will have progressed to be invasive. Usually, if the recurrence occurs after excision and radiation therapy for the initial cancer, a total mastectomy is necessary.

With careful attention to the type and extent of DCIS, the use of partial mastectomy plus radiation therapy, and regular follow up with mammograms, the cure rate should be equal to the cure rate with mastectomy.

If the ductal carcinoma in situ is extensive

If the in situ cancer is widespread (more than 5 cm across or involving more than one-quarter of the breast), the amount of tissue that must be removed often leads to unacceptable disfigurement of the breast. Also, even if an extensive area of DCIS can be satisfactorily removed and the patient receives radiation therapy there may be a high (30 to 40%) chance of recurrence in the breast. Since about half of these recurrences will be invasive, when the in situ cancer is very extensive, total mastectomy with or without immediate reconstruction is usually recommended to maximize the chances of long-term cure.

Wide excision alone for very small DCIS

For some women with relatively small areas of DCIS, it may be possible to save the breast and avoid radiation therapy. For this approach to be successful, the cancer should be less than 1.5 cm in diameter on both the mammogram and pathology, *and* the cancer should not be the high-grade subtype (very abnormal-looking cells with necrosis) *and* to be confidant that the DCIS has been completely removed, there should be at least 1 cm of normal breast tissue between any ducts containing DCIS and the edge of the excision specimen. Radiation therapy will still reduce the risk of breast recurrence further, but because the risk of recurrence is relatively low with surgery alone in these cases, only a few women among every hundred treated would benefit from the radiation therapy. Research in this area is ongoing.

High-grade ductal carcinoma in situ

Ductal carcinoma in situ that has very abnormal-appearing cells (Grade 3; see Chapter 14) and a lot of necrosis in the milk ducts tends to develop recurrences more often than the other types of in situ cancer and also tends to form invasive cancers earlier. These types of lesions are sometimes called *comedocarcinoma*. To achieve the best control, some authorities recommend adding radiation after wide excision for any size of comedocarcinoma, even if it is very small.

The boxed information at the end of this chapter summarizes recommendations for the management of ductal carcinoma in situ.

Tamoxifen and other hormonal therapy

Tamoxifen, at a dose of 20 mg per day for 5 years, can decrease both the recurrence of in situ cancer and the development of invasive breast cancer. Tamoxifen may be particularly helpful if the DCIS was estrogen-receptor positive. Tamoxifen may also decrease the chance of developing cancer in the opposite breast. However, studies to date suggest that overall survival, 10 years after the initial diagnosis and treatment of a DCIS was equal, regardless of whether or not women received tamoxifen.

Tamoxifen may cause side effects, including hot flushes, mood disturbance (depression), a small risk of endometrial cancer, and an increased risk of thrombosis (blood clots). Therefore, before taking tamoxifen, women with DCIS should carefully balance the risk of cancer recurrence with the risk of serious side effects before making a decision about taking the drug. Women who have had bilateral mastectomies (both breasts removed) and are not at risk of further local disease, or have a history of blood clots, or have other severe health problems or advanced age and are unlikely to live another 10 years, will not benefit sufficiently from tamoxifen to outweigh the side effects.

In recent years there have been several studies that have shown that aromatase inhibitors (see Chapter 27), used on their own or following several years of tamoxifen, have a greater ability to reduce breast cancer recurrence compared to using tamoxifen alone. All those studies involved patients with invasive breast cancer. Current studies are examining the role of aromatase inhibitors in postmenopausal women with DCIS and as a breast cancer prevention agent. However, aromatase inhibitors are not currently recommended as treatment for patients with DCIS.

Options for treatment of the breast with DCIS

Wide excision (partial mastectomy) alone is appropriate if:
- The cancer is less than 1.5 cm *and*
- Not a high grade subtype *and*
- A good margin (1 cm or more) of normal breast tissue was seen between the cancer and the edge of the surgical specimen

Wide excision (partial mastectomy) plus radiation therapy is appropriate if:
- The cancer is less than 5 cm in diameter *or*
- Was the Grade 3 subtype *or*
- The margin between the DCIS and the edge of the removed tissue is less than 1 cm
- An option for any size or type of DCIS

Total mastectomy is appropriate if:
- The cancer is extensive (more than 5 cm in diameter on pathology or the width of calcifications on a mammogram) *or*
- The margins still show cancer after two attempts at wide excision *or*
- The patient chooses this option for any size or type of in situ cancer

---

Treatment of lobular carcinoma in situ

Women with lobular carcinoma in situ (LCIS, also called *intra-epithelial lobular neoplasia*) have a higher-than-average risk of developing an invasive breast cancer some time in the future. Over-all, the chance of developing breast cancer is about 20 to 30% over the next 20 years. The risk of developing invasive breast cancer is related to the extent of LCIS. If there are just focal deposits, the risk is not much higher than for an average woman of the same age. If the LCIS is very extensive, the risk of subsequent cancer may be from four to 10 times higher than for a woman without LCIS. The invasive cancers are about as likely to develop in either breast, so therapy or surveillance has to be directed at both breasts.

One course of action is to undertake careful, regular screening and follow-up. Another, drastic choice that has been used is preventive removal of both breasts (bilateral prophylactic mastectomy; see Chapter 19 on total mastectomy). This is only done on rare occasions when a woman's fear of developing breast cancer outweighs her desire to save her breasts. This surgery may be recommended if a woman with lobular carcinoma in situ also has a strong family history of breast cancer.

Lobular cancers are almost always estrogen receptor-positive (see Chapter 27), which suggests that the anti-estrogen drug tamoxifen might be able to block the stimulating effect of natural estrogens and help prevent the development of invasive cancers. A large study demonstrated that for women with LCIS, tamoxifen reduced the chance of developing an invasive breast cancer. Although tamoxifen is usually well tolerated, it does have some potentially serious side effects such as blood clots in the legs and lungs and a higher risk of developing cancer of the uterus. In addition, tamoxifen can affect one's quality of life by causing hot flushes, vaginal dryness, and depression.

Because of the potential serious side effects, it is not clear whether all women with LCIS should take tamoxifen to prevent the development of breast cancer. Each woman needs to consider other options as well as take into account her individual likelihood of developing invasive cancer (age, family history, extensiveness of the LCIS) and her general health (tamoxifen should not be taken if a woman had phlebitis or blood clots in the past). Women with a family history of breast cancer, extensive LCIS, and no history of phlebitis may benefit sufficiently from tamoxifen to warrant taking it for 5 years.

Radiation therapy

CHAPTER TWENTY-FOUR

Radiation therapy: What is it?

How does radiation work?

RADIATION THERAPY, ALSO CALLED *radiotherapy*, is the use of high-energy rays to kill cancer cells. Radiation works by damaging cells so that they eventually die. Radiation will damage any type of cell, either normal or cancerous, so great care must be taken during the planning and delivery of the radiation therapy so that as much healthy tissue as possible can be avoided.

Fortunately, normal cells repair themselves from radiation damage more completely than cancer cells do. By giving the radiation in a series of small treatments, once or sometimes twice a day, normal cells have a chance to recover between treatments while the cancer cells die.

When is radiation given?

Radiation therapy is useful in helping prevent regrowth or progression of cancer in the part of the body that is treated, for example the breast, chest wall, or lymph nodes. After a lumpectomy, radiation is directed at the breast to kill any possible remaining cancer cells. It may also be used to treat cancer that has spread beyond the breast or lymph nodes. For example, if breast cancer has spread to a woman's hip bone and is causing pain, radiation to the hip may kill the cancer cells there and relieve the pain.

The benefits and side effects of radiation therapy are generally restricted to the area being treated. In contrast, chemotherapy and hormonal therapy drugs are absorbed into the blood stream and affect many parts of the body.

The procedure for getting radiotherapy

The process can be considered in three steps:
1. Deciding whether treatment is advisable.
2. Attending a planning visit in the radiation department where the area of treatment will be identified, marked, and measurements will be taken to calculate the radiation dose.
3. Receiving radiotherapy during daily visits according to a planned schedule.

The treatment decision

You make the decision to proceed with radiotherapy in consultation with a radiation oncologist (a specialist in radiation therapy). The issues to consider are described in Chapter 25.

The planning session

The purpose of this session is to map out exactly how the radiation therapy will be directed, given your individual size and body shape, and the part of the body that requires treatment. Very specific information, such as your body and arm position, is recorded during the planning session so that you will be set up accurately each day during the actual radiation treatment.

The area to be treated is usually marked out using a machine called a simulator. The simulator sends low-energy X-rays through the body onto a screen or film so that the target area to be treated can be determined exactly. Usually a CT-simulator is used. The CT is a large, donut-shaped machine. The patient lies on a table and is moved through the hole in the donut while X-rays are taken. The CT produces a cross-sectional image, for example of the breast and internal anatomy of the chest (Figure 21). The CT makes it easier for the radiation oncologist to design a treatment plan that includes all of the necessary tissue but excludes from the radiation beam as much normal tissue as possible, for instance the heart and lung during treatment of the left breast.

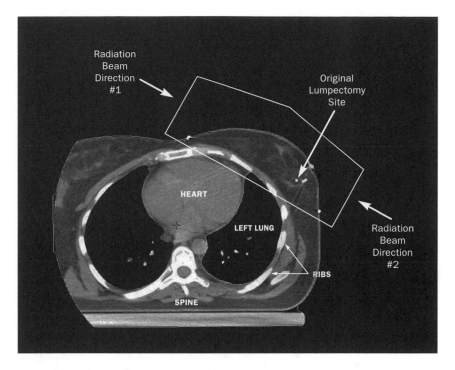

Figure 21: A radiation-planning CT scan through the breast showing the organs nearby that are at risk of side effects from radiation, the lungs, heart, ribs, and skin. The original lumpectomy site in the left breast is marked. Radiation is directed through the breast from side to side and is angled to avoid as much lung and heart tissue as possible.

Two to four permanent ink dots, the size of a small freckle, are often placed at the centre or corner of the treatment area. These dots are reference points used for the daily treatments and can be useful if radiation is being considered again sometime in the future. Sometimes temporary ink marks are also placed on the skin to help with daily treatment set-ups.

Treatment sessions

The amount of radiation you receive and the number of daily visits depends on the amount of tissue to be treated, and whether the goal of treatment is to treat a mass of cancer, prevent a recurrence after surgery, or to relieve symptoms. Usually, adjuvant or curative radiation therapy requires from 3 to 6 weeks of daily treatments. When the goal is symptom relief, a single treatment or 1 to 3 weeks of treatment is usually sufficient.

What happens during radiation treatment?

Radiation therapy is most often delivered using a large machine called a *linear accelerator*. Radiation treatments are painless. In fact, when the machine is on, the only thing you'll notice is a slight whirring sound. Treatments may be given from several angles each day (Figure 22).

You will be in the treatment room for about 10 to 20 minutes. Most of this time is spent carefully adjusting the treatment machine so that it is positioned correctly each day. During a typical treatment session the machine is turned on for only 1 to 3 minutes per treated area each day.

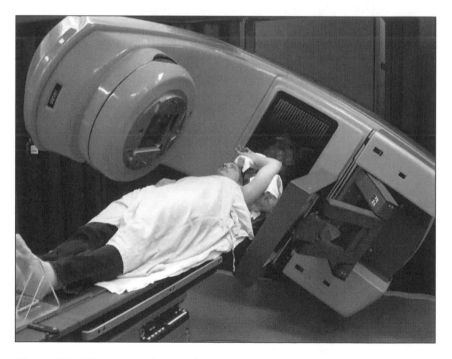

Figure 22: Woman getting ready for treatment on a radiotherapy machine.

How much radiation is given during radiotherapy?

The amount of radiation given is limited by the amount the normal tissues can tolerate. The basic unit of radiation dose is called a Gray. The amount of radiation received during a chest X-ray is approximately 0.005 Gray. For a mammogram it is 0.003 Gray. In contrast, the typical total dose used to treat the whole breast during cancer therapy ranges from 40 Gray (divided into 15 daily doses given over 3 weeks) up to 50 Gray (divided into 25 daily doses given over 5 weeks). If only a part of the breast is being treated (see Chapter 25), the dose of radiation varies considerably with the partial breast radiation technique that is used and whether it is done as a single treatment during the lumpectomy or as a week of treatment after surgery.

Brachytherapy—a way to give partial breast radiation therapy

In brachytherapy, instead of using a machine that sends out an X-ray beam, a tiny piece of radioactive material is implanted directly into a tumour or into the area from which the tumour was removed. Radioactive iridium is the substance most often used for brachytherapy, but other materials such as radioactive gold or palladium are also used.

Under local or general anaesthetic, hollow tubes are placed into the breast around the surgical site. These are stitched into place. This is called the *implant*. Later, in the clinic, the doctor or technician places the radioactive material into the tubes, usually with a remotely controlled device. Treatments may be given twice a day for a week. The patient has the tubes in her breast for the week but she is not radioactive when she goes home.

Depending on the radioactive material used and the dose, the radiation sources may be left in place continuously or may be inserted into the implant tubes once or twice a day for several days. During active treatment, the hospital room is considered to be radioactive and visitors are restricted.

An experimental form of brachytherapy that is gaining popularity uses a permanent implant. In this technique, up to 100 radioactive pellets the size of an uncooked grain of rice are inserted into the breast tissue surrounding the lumpectomy site. These radioactive "seeds" are left in the breast permanently. The side effects and benefits of this technique are being tested in a research study involving women with very small tumours that appear to have been completely removed and who do not have any cancer spread to the axilla (armpit) lymph nodes.

Can radiation be repeated at some time in the future?

When giving radiation therapy to a part of the body, the idea is to maximize the destruction of the cancer while staying within safe limits of the normal surrounding tissues. If a part of the body has already received the maximum safe radiation dose it is usually not possible to re-treat that area. Occasionally, if a fairly low dose of radiation was used and cancer regrowth causes symptoms at the same site, the area can be re-treated. If an entirely new area of the body develops problems from cancer, radiation therapy can generally be safely delivered to the new area.

CHAPTER TWENTY-FIVE

Who benefits from radiation therapy?

THERE ARE FOUR GENERAL SITUATIONS in which radiotherapy is used for women with breast cancer:
- After a breast-saving partial mastectomy
- After a modified radical mastectomy when there is a high chance of recurrence on the chest wall or in the lymph nodes
- As treatment for locally advanced cancer when surgery is not advisable
- For the relief of symptoms due to cancer recurrence on the chest wall or metastases to other part of the body such as the bones, lymph nodes, or the brain

Radiotherapy following lumpectomy or partial mastectomy

Research studies from Canada, the US, and Europe have shown that giving radiation after a lumpectomy substantially reduces the chance that cancer will regrow in the breast. Preventing cancer regrowth in the breast also improves survival by several percent.

Even when it appears that the entire tumour has been removed, studies have shown that there is still a risk of cancer regrowing in the breast, and having a course of radiation therapy after the partial mastectomy reduces this risk. The cancer regrows from a small number of cancer cells that may extend several centimetres from the original tumour location. For this reason, usually the entire breast is treated with radiation.

During radiation therapy to the breast, the treatment is delivered from side to side across the breast to reduce, as much as possible, treatment of normal structures inside the chest such as the lung or heart (Figure 21, page 143). Careful planning of the radiation therapy, including the use of a CT scanner, helps prevent side effects. Women with cancer spread to the axillary lymph nodes may also receive radiotherapy to the lymph node regions above and below the collarbone (see below).

In some circumstances, an additional amount of radiation, called a *boost*, may be given to the surgery site. The boost often takes an additional 1 to 2 weeks of treatment visits. A boost reduces the risk of local recurrence and is given if the risk of re-growth in the breast is higher than average. Women younger than age 50 or who have cancer very close or at the edge of the tissue removed at surgery have a higher risk of breast cancer recurrence and are often given an additional boost dose of radiation.

Partial breast radiation: Is it safe and effective?

Follow-up of women treated with lumpectomy has shown that if cancer regrows in the breast, 70 to 80% of the time, it is within a few centimetres (less than 1 inch) from the original surgery site. Exceptions are women with diffuse ductal carcinoma in situ, women who had more than one cancer in the breast, those whose cancer had spread to the lymph nodes, or women whose tumour was of the lobular type (see Chapter 14).

The potential advantages of partial breast radiation are that a smaller part of the body is treated with less normal tissue exposed to radiation, and that the treatment is more convenient because it can often be completed in a single treatment or 1 week rather than the 3 to 6 weeks that are customary with whole breast radiation therapy. Partial breast radiation may be done with standard radiation machines, with brachytherapy or by delivering a single large dose of radiation at the time of lumpectomy with a special machine installed in the operating room.

There are two potential concerns with partial breast radiation. One is that there may be a higher risk of cancer regrowth in the parts of the breast that were not treated with radiation. The other concern is that the higher daily doses of radiation that are used to shorten the treatment to just 1 week may result in more scarring or thickening of the breast tissue around the surgical site. Research is ongoing to determine if partial breast radiation therapy is as safe and effective as whole breast radiation therapy after a lumpectomy.

Radiotherapy after modified radical mastectomy

Total mastectomy (complete removal of the breast) without radiotherapy achieves local control of breast cancer for most patients with stage I or II breast cancer. However, depending on the extent and type of cancer, the risk of regrowth on the chest wall or in the lymph nodes can be particularly high and radiation may be recommended after mastectomy. Radiation is usually recommended if the cancer was larger than 5 cm, had invaded the adjacent skin or chest wall muscles, or showed extensive spread to the lymph nodes. In these circumstances, the risk of regrowth is usually greater than 30% and the use of radiation therapy may reduce the chance of regrowth to less than 10%.

Until the mid-1990s it was thought that radiation did not improve survival. However, long-term follow-up of research studies comparing radiation to no radiation after mastectomy have demonstrated that radiation added after mastectomy improves survival for some patients. In the research studies involving women with cancer spread to their lymph nodes, 5 to 8% more women who received radiation therapy after their mastectomy were alive, free of breast cancer 10 to 15 years later. This benefit must be balanced against an increased risk of side effects (see Chapter 26).

There are differing opinions regarding whether *all* women with cancer spread to their lymph nodes should have radiation to the chest wall and lymph node regions or whether the radiation should just be used for women with higher risk disease, for example with more than three lymph nodes affected with cancer. Balancing the potential benefits with the risk of increased long-term side effects requires consideration of the characteristics and extent of the cancer in the breast and axilla, the woman's current health, the extent of axillary surgery done, and whether there are any signs of arm swelling or other complications after the surgery. The more extensive the cancer and the greater the number of cancer-involved lymph nodes, the more worthwhile it is to have radiation therapy. For patients with one to three lymph nodes containing cancer, additional factors such as the presence of Grade 3 disease, cancer found in the lymphatic channels or blood vessels in the breast (see Chapter 12) and young age of the patient can identify women at higher risk of cancer regrowth and therefore patients likely to receive a larger benefit from the radiation therapy.

One also needs to consider the extent of surgery. If more than 10 to 15 lymph nodes were removed or if the woman already has some arm or hand swelling or a history of heart of lung problems, the chance of serious side effects from the radiation may outweigh the benefits. Women with cancer spread to their lymph nodes should expect to discuss these issues with their radiation oncologist. Whether to use radiation to the regional nodes in addition to chemotherapy, Herceptin, and hormone treatments is a particularly difficult balance for women with only small amounts of disease in their axillary lymph nodes.

Radiotherapy for locally extensive cancer

At the time of diagnosis some women already have a cancer that is considered too extensive to treat with surgery. In other cases, a woman may not be fit for surgery. These women usually receive chemotherapy or hormone therapy depending on their tumour type, age, and fitness to withstand treatment. In addition they usually receive radiation to the breast and the nearby lymph nodes. As a result of these treatments, the cancer may shrink to a size that makes surgery possible.

Radiotherapy for recurrence and relief of symptoms from metastases

Radiotherapy can be especially useful to improve the quality of life of patients who have recurrent cancer or who suffer from symptoms caused by cancer that has spread to other areas of the body (metastases). In these situations, the radiation works by killing cancer cells, thereby shrinking the cancer lumps and relieving pain or other symptoms. Pain caused by breast cancer metastases to the bones can be relieved in approximately 75% of cases. When there are metastases in the brain, lymph nodes near the breast or some other sites, improvement of symptoms occurs in about 50% of patients who receive radiation therapy. To treat metastatic cancer, radiation therapy is usually given as a single treatment or 1 week of treatment.

Radiotherapy is not usually used when the cancer has spread to the lung tissue or the liver because the dose of radiation necessary to kill the cancer cells in these areas is too high for the organs to tolerate. In these situations, hormones or chemotherapy (or both) may be used (see Chapter 39).

CHAPTER TWENTY-SIX

Side effects of radiation therapy

What radiotherapy does not cause

RADIATION TREATMENTS THEMSELVES are usually painless. Some people may experience nausea if a very large area of the body is treated. You will not lose your hair unless the radiation is specifically directed at your head. Except when brachytherapy is used (insertion of radiation sources directly into the breast, see Chapter 24), you are *not* radioactive and you are not a threat to your friends, family, or pets. Radiation does not make you dizzy or lightheaded. You should feel well enough to drive yourself back and forth to the cancer centre for your treatments. Some women even continue full-time employment during radiation treatment.

You may feel tired

The response to radiation is quite variable but most people experience some fatigue. About one woman in three will become noticeably tired. The cause is not known, but the best remedy is to have an afternoon nap, maintain a balanced diet, and cut back on stressful activities. After the radiation treatment is finished, the fatigue decreases gradually over several weeks or months but some women find they have noticeable fatigue for a year. It is often difficult to tell whether the fatigue is due to the effects of the treatment or the psychological and emotional stress and the life disruption that a new diagnosis of breast cancer brings to every woman.

Emotional effects

Another effect of going to radiation therapy sessions is the daily reminder of the cancer. Many women report that they feel weepy, depressed, angry, or frustrated. Discuss your feelings with your radiation therapist and oncologist. You will find that it is a normal, common reaction. Your sense of frustration could be relieved by asserting some control over the process by altering the timing of your appointments to suit you better or simply by expressing concerns and asking questions.

Side effects in the treated breast

The skin

After a partial mastectomy, it is usual for the entire breast, skin, and chest wall underneath to be treated with radiation. During several weeks of treatment, the skin gradually becomes pink, red, or sun burnt and may eventually peel. Afterwards, the skin may appear tanned. The redness or tanning usually disappears slowly but some women are left with slightly darker skin on a permanent basis. Occasionally the skin may blister, usually around the nipple, in the armpit area, or in the crease beneath the breast. Over time the areola on the treated breast may become pale.

Toward the end of a course of radiation therapy the skin tends to become dry and this causes itchiness. In the past, women were told to keep the skin dry with a dusting of cornstarch. Today it is recognized that the skin feels much better and radiation reactions are actually reduced if the skin is kept moist. It is recommended that you apply a moisturizing cream two to three times a day during radiation unless the skin breaks down. A hydrocortisone cream can also reduce the sense of burning as the radiation reaction builds up. If the skin cracks or blisters, it is often helpful to apply a commercial antibiotic cream such as Flamazine (silver sulfadiazine) unless you are allergic to sulfa drugs. If the skin has a severe or painful reaction or breaks down, you should speak to your radiation therapist or nurse for additional advice or treatment.

The radiation reaction in the skin is often maximal about 1 to 2 weeks after the radiation treatment is finished. Continued use of a moisturizing cream will reduce the itching and help to lift off any dead or peeling skin, especially around the nipple, which may remain crusty for several months.

Breast firmness and tenderness

You may notice that the treated breast is slightly firmer than the untreated one. Radiation can cause the breast to become enlarged, tender, or heavy with fluid during treatment. This may last for 6 to 18 months afterwards. This is particularly a problem if the breast is swollen, red, infected, or heavily bruised from the surgery. To improve comfort during and after radiation therapy, it is advised that you wear a bra that is supportive and nonconstricting. Don't wear a bra that leaves indentations in the breast. The most comfortable bra is often a cotton sport bra without much elastic material and without lace or seams.

Approximately 25% of women will have some mild to moderate discomfort in the rib cage even years after radiation, and feel more tenderness if bumped on the treated side.

Rarely, radiation may cause severe scarring and fibrosis, with discomfort and deformity of the breast. Women who have a lot of swelling, bruising, or infection of the breast after surgery are more prone to develop permanent scarring. A small percentage of women (less than 1%) will develop significant scarring and permanent breast hardness for no known reason.

Electric shock sensations and prominent blood vessels

It is normal to experience occasional sharp "electric shock" sensations in the breast or chest wall. This is not a sign of cancer. These fleeting pains are from nerves, damaged during surgery, trying to repair themselves. It is common, even years after treatment, for the treated breast to be a bit tender or more sensitive (for example, if bumped) than the other breast. A small percentage of women may have prolonged breast tenderness requiring pain killers.

Red "spidery" blood vessels may appear 18 to 24 months or more after treatment. This is called *telangiectasia*. While potentially unsightly, these are *not* a sign of cancer.

Side effects of treating the lymph node regions

The throat

If the lymph nodes near the collarbone are treated, part of the throat and the top of the lung will be in the path of the radiation beam. You may experience a temporary sore or scratchy throat or the feeling of a lump in the throat. These symptoms are *not* due to cancer, they are just part of the treatment.

The lungs

Sometimes the lung becomes inflamed a few weeks to several months after the radiation treatment. This reaction is called *radiation pneumonitis*. If you develop this condition, you will experience a dry, persistent cough, fatigue, and, in some cases, fever and chest pain. The pneumonitis usually clears by itself after 3 to 6 months, but treatment with steroids may improve symptoms if they are severe.

The heart

The heart is located inside the chest behind the left breast. Sometimes, especially when the lymph nodes are included in the radiation volume, a small part of the heart may receive radiation therapy. If this happens, the radiation may accelerate hardening of the arteries in the heart. Some studies of women treated with older radiation therapy techniques and who lived 15 or more years after breast cancer treatment, have shown that women treated with radiation for left-sided breast cancer have a small (about 1%) increased chance of having a heart attack. Considerable effort is made during the planning of the radiation therapy to exclude the heart from the radiation beam.

Scarring under the arm

Radiation may increase the amount of scarring caused by surgery in the axilla (armpit). In turn, this may cause scarring in the lymphatic channels and increase the chance of developing arm swelling. It is important to work at regaining full use of your shoulder if a full axillary dissection was performed. To reduce the chance of developing lymphedema, it is important, on a permanent basis, to pay careful attention to hand and arm care and to avoid cuts, burns, and infections in the hand or arm.

Scarring of the chest wall

If radiation is given to the chest wall after mastectomy it can cause some firmness and scarring in the skin and underlying tissues. Approximately 25% of women will have some mild to moderate discomfort in the rib cage even years after radiation, and feel more tenderness if bumped on the treated side. Rarely, radiation may cause a rib to crack or break. If radiation is given after reconstruction with a breast prostheses (Chapter 34), there is a greater chance of scarring around the prosthesis. This may make the breast mound hard and it can retract up the chest wall toward the collarbone.

Does radiation therapy itself cause cancer?

Low doses of radiation may cause cancer, especially in people younger than age 20. However, the high doses used for breast cancer therapy have a low risk of causing cancer. An uncommon form of skin cancer called an *angiosarcoma* has been reported to develop in the treatment area in approximately one in every 1,000 women who survive more than 10 years after initially being treated for breast cancer. This risk needs to be compared to the chance that radiation will prevent the re-growth of the breast cancer—often 100 to 200 women per 1,000 receiving radiation will benefit by avoiding regrowth of the known breast cancer. There is conflicting evidence about whether radiation therapy for breast cancer increases the risk of other cancers but some studies have shown a small increased risk of lung cancer in women surviving 10 to 20 years after the treatment.

Hormone therapy

CHAPTER TWENTY-SEVEN

Hormone therapy:
What is it and who benefits from it?

What are the female hormones?

THE FEMALE HORMONES estrogen and progesterone control many of the female and sex-related processes of the body, such as the growth of female genitals and breasts, development of the female body shape, and regulation of the menstrual cycle.

What is the relationship between hormones and breast cancer?

Estrogen not only stimulates the growth of the breasts but also appears to encourage the growth of some, but not all, breast cancers. Progesterone can also simulate the growth of breast tumours.

Hormone receptors in the tumour determine if hormone therapy will be effective

Hormone treatment (also known as *endocrine treatment*) is only effective in tumours that have hormone receptors (see Chapter 14). For patients with hormone receptor-positive tumours, endocrine therapy is often the most effective and most important drug treatment. Hormone receptors can be either estrogen receptors (ER) or progesterone receptors (PR) and are found in approximately 70% of breast cancers. They are measured in the tumour by the pathologist and predict if the tumour will respond to hormone treatment. Most laboratories use an immunohistochemical method to measure the amount of receptor in a particular cancer as 0, 1+, 2+, or 3+, where 0 is negative for receptors and 3+ is a high receptor content. In general the higher the estrogen receptor content in the tumour, the more responsive the tumour will be to hormone treatments. Many laboratories use the Allred rating scale to report the degree of receptor activity from 0 to 8, with 8 being very high and less than 3 being negative.

ER or PR: Are they both important?

Estrogen receptors are more frequent and appear to be the more important receptor. Progesterone receptors appear to generally affect how well the estrogen receptor functions. Tumours may have both receptors positive (ER+PR+), just estrogen receptors positive (ER+PR-) or both negative (ER-PR-). With current pathology methods it is very rare to find tumours that are ER-PR+.

What is hormone therapy?

Hormone therapy for breast cancer (sometimes called *anti-estrogen therapy*) is a form of whole body treatment that is used as adjuvant treatment or for cancer recurrence. The term *hormone therapy* refers to a number of different treatments designed to affect the level of female hormones in the body. These include the use of drugs for both premenopausal and postmenopausal women or the removal or destruction of the ovaries in premenopausal women by surgery, medications, or radiation.

Changing the hormone levels in the body affects receptor-positive cancer cells and slows their growth. A number of different drugs can do this effectively. The particular drug chosen depends on whether the woman is premenopausal or postmenopausal and the stage of her disease since not all drugs have been proven to be effective for all stages. Hormone therapy is used for prevention, in situ disease, as neoadjuvant (prior to surgery) or adjuvant therapy of invasive disease, and in recurrent breast cancer. Hormone therapy has been shown to decrease the chance of the cancer coming back both in the affected breast and in the rest of the body, and also has been shown to decrease the risk of a new cancer developing in the opposite breast.

A woman with breast cancer is defined as premenopausal or postmenopausal based on whether she had a menstrual cycle in the year prior to the time of treatment. This chapter will focus on general hormone therapy recommendations after surgery. Chapter 28 will discuss side effects.

Hormone therapy in premenopausal women

Before menopause, estrogen is made primarily by the ovaries. The pituitary gland, which is in the brain, releases hormones (LH and FSH) that control ovulation, the menstrual cycle, and the production of estrogen in the ovaries. Pituitary gland hormones are released based on the level of estrogen in the blood. When the estrogen level goes down FSH is released to stimulate the ovaries. Pituitary hormones are also released at different times during the menstrual cycle. Regular menstrual cycles are a sign of normal ovarian function but do not tell the whole story. Many women's periods get irregular or stop with chemotherapy. But sometimes ovarian function returns and the ovaries are still able to produce estrogen.

The goal of hormone therapy in premenopausal women with breast cancer is to either stop the production of estrogen or block the effect of the estrogen on the breast cancer cells.

Tamoxifen

Tamoxifen (Novaldex, Tamofen, etc.) is effective in stopping the effect of estrogen on the breast cancer cells. Tamoxifen has been shown to be effective in the adjuvant therapy of both in situ and invasive cancers that have hormone receptors. The decision to use tamoxifen as adjuvant therapy is based on the risk of the cancer recurring. This risk is based primarily on the size of the tumour, the involvement of axillary nodes, the grade, the finding of lymphatic or vascular invasion, and the hormone receptor status.

Tamoxifen is a "prodrug," meaning it is inactive when introduced to the body, but changed into an active drug, endoxifen, by the body's enzymes, including one named Cyp2D6. Women can be classified into three groups by measuring Cyp2D6 levels in the blood. Although some studies suggested that such a classification would help predict response to tamoxifen, more recent studies have not shown a correlation. At this time checking Cyp2D6 levels prior to starting tamoxifen is not recommended.

Ovarian suppression

Since the ovaries produce estrogen in premenopausal women, suppressing the ovaries will decrease the estrogen levels. This has been shown to be an effective breast cancer treatment in premenopausal women with estrogen-responsive tumours. Ovarian hormone production can be stopped with surgery (oophorectomy), radiation therapy, or drug therapy (see Chapter 28).

Oophorectomy

Oophorectomy is the surgical removal of the ovaries, which can be done with minimal surgery (laparoscopically) or with a full surgical procedure with or without the removal of the uterus. Removing the uterus does not affect the estrogen levels.

Radiation

Radiation directed to the ovaries, usually once per day for 5 days, damages the ovaries sufficiently that they stop producing estrogens. It generally takes about 3 months after radiation to decrease the levels of estrogen to a postmenopausal level.

Pituitary suppression

Drugs called *LHRH-agonists* interfere with the normal pathway of the pituitary hormones, LH and FSH. By blocking the release of LH and FSH, the ovaries temporarily stop producing estrogen. When the drugs are stopped, the ovaries generally start working normally again. LHRH-agonists are given as an intramuscular injection every month or once every 3 months for 2 to 5 years when used as adjuvant treatment. These drugs include goserelin (Zoladex), buserelin (Suprefact), triptorelin (Trelstar), and leuprolide (Lupron). The LHRH-agonists are usually given with an oral hormone treatment.

Hormone therapy in postmenopausal women

A woman is defined as postmenopausal when she has not had periods for a year. Women who have had their uterus removed (hysterectomy) but still have their ovaries are not postmenopausal until their ovaries stop producing estrogen. Menopause may be suspected if the woman has menopausal symptoms such as hot flushes and can be confirmed by a blood test for hormone levels. The average age of menopause in North America is 52 years. Since some women experience symptoms of hot flushes, vaginal dryness, mood changes, an increased risk of osteoporosis, and skin changes, menopause is often discussed as if it were a disease when in fact, it is simply a normal physiological event.

After menopause, a woman still makes estrogen but the levels of estrogen are significantly lower than before menopause. The body makes estrogen by a complicated process that involves the adrenal glands, their production of cholesterol, and its eventual change into estrogen. The last enzyme involved in this long process of converting cholesterol to estrogen is called *aromatase*. The aromatase enzyme is found in a large number of tissues in the body including fat, muscle, liver, breast, and breast cancer cells.

In postmenopausal women, hormone-sensitive breast cancers can be treated either by blocking the estrogen receptor on the cell (tamoxifen) or by interfering with the aromatase enzyme to stop estrogen production. The later is accomplished by a group of drugs known as aromatase inhibitors: anastrozole (Arimidex), letrozole (Femara) and exemestane (Aromasin).

Tamoxifen

As well as decreasing the risk of cancer recurrence (see above), tamoxifen may have other beneficial effects for postmenopausal women. It reduces cholesterol and lipids in the blood, which may be good for the heart. Some studies have also shown that women who took tamoxifen had less calcium loss from their bones, fewer fractures, and less osteoporosis.

Aromatase inhibitors

The aromatase inhibitors act by blocking the enzyme aromatase and are only effective in women who are truly postmenopausal and not making estrogen in their ovaries.

Anastrozole (Arimidex), letrozole (Femara) and exemestane (Aromasin) have all been shown to be effective in early breast cancer by decreasing the chance of the cancer regrowing in the affected breast or elsewhere in the body and by decreasing the chance of a new cancer growing in the other breast. There is also evidence that exemestane can reduce the chance of developing breast cancer when taken by women at high risk of developing breast cancer. Various studies have been conducted using these drugs instead of tamoxifen, after 2 to 3 years of tamoxifen for another 2 to 3 years to make up a total of 5 years and in the case of letrozole, after completing 5 years of tamoxifen. Ongoing research studies will add to and refine our knowledge of how to best use the aromatase inhibitors. However, if a woman is postmenopausal and has a hormone receptor-positive tumour, these drugs should be discussed as an option for adjuvant treatment.

Two studies have reported that longer hormone adjuvant therapy may be helpful. The first and largest study was the MA17 study that added letrozole after 5 years of tamoxifen. The MA17 study showed that women had fewer recurrences by taking the aromatase inhibitor after completing 5 years of tamoxifen. Women completing 5 years of tamoxifen should discuss the use of letrozole with their doctors and decide whether to take it based on the risk of the initial tumour and other health problems. As well, two studies, the ATLAS and ATTOM studies, have suggested that taking more then 5 years of tamoxifen may be helpful. These studies contradict others that suggested that taking more than 5 years of tamoxifen was not helpful. A full report of these studies has not been published, so at this time, taking more than 5 years of tamoxifen is not recommended. There are studies ongoing to see if after 3 to 5 years of an aromatase inhibitor more treatment is effective, but these have not been published yet.

Chapter Twenty-Eight

Side effects of hormone therapy

Do hormone therapies have side effects?

As with all drug treatments, there are potential side effects associated with hormone treatments but this must be balanced with the benefit from the treatment. The side effects may depend on the drug but they also vary significantly between individuals. Some women have no side effects while others suffer with many.

Menopausal symptoms

Any drug that either causes menopause to occur (LHRH agonists, see Chapter 27) or that lowers estrogen (aromatase inhibitors) can cause the symptoms associated with low body levels of estrogen. Not all women experience symptoms with menopause. Sometimes symptoms are more severe if a woman experiences a sudden decrease in the estrogen level, as happens when a woman has her ovaries removed, stops estrogen replacement therapy, or goes into menopause with chemotherapy.

Hot flushes

Hot flushes may be minor or may be severe. They are often temporary and most women report they get better with time. Avoiding triggers such a caffeine (found in coffee, tea, chocolate, and colas), alcohol, and stress may be beneficial. Plant estrogens such as black cohosh may be helpful, but it is not clear if they (or soy) have sufficient estrogen effects to act on breast cancer cells and should probably be used in the lowest dose to help symptoms and for a limited time. Prescription medications including low doses of anti-depressants such as Effexor (venlafaxine), and the nerve blocker gabapentin have been shown to reduce the number and severity of hot flushes, as has the drug Dixarit (clonidine).

Vaginal dryness and irritation

Vaginal dryness and irritation can make sexual intercourse painful and difficult. Lubricating gels such as Replens, Muko, Astroglide, or Slippery Stuff may be helpful. Lubricants can be applied to the vaginal opening and the head of the penis to make intercourse easier. If the symptoms are severe, it is sometimes helpful to use a small amount of estrogen. This may be in the form of an estrogen cream or intravaginal estrogens such as Vagi-Fems or Estring. Estring is an intravaginal ring that slowly releases a low dose of estrogen into the vagina and may decrease dryness and irritation. Although some of the estrogen may be released into the blood stream, the amount is so small that the risk is likely minimal. However there are concerns, particularly with the aromatase inhibitors, that the estrogen may decrease the effect of the anti-cancer treatment. There is less concern in using vaginal estrogens with tamoxifen because its mechanism of action is different than the aromatase inhibitors. The improved quality of life from using small amounts of vaginal estrogens may be more important to some women than a theoretical and small decreased effectiveness of the tamoxifen or aromatase inhibitors. The potential risks and benefits of vaginal estrogen treatment should be discussed with your doctor if vaginal dryness or irritation is a problem.

Osteoporosis and increased risk of fractures

Without estrogen there is a loss of calcium from the bones and the risk of bone fractures and osteoporosis increase. Women who have a family history of osteoporosis, who smoke, drink excessive coffee or alcohol, or who have been on medications such as steroids for a long time have an increased risk of osteoporosis. It is recommended that all premenopausal women take 1000 mg of calcium and 1000 IU or more of vitamin D per day and that postmenopausal women ingest 1500 mg of calcium and 800 IU of vitamin D per day. Chapter 35 lists foods that contain calcium. It is helpful to look at your usual diet and calculate approximately how much calcium and vitamin D you need to take as a calcium supplement. Regular weight-bearing exercise is also important to bone health. For women taking an aromatase inhibitor, a baseline bone density should be done and repeated every 24 months. If there is significant bone loss, these drugs may not be appropriate and treatment with a medication to improve bone density (possibly a bisphosphanate) may be indicated.

Weight gain

Many women gain a few kilograms at the time of menopause. This may also occur if one is taking hormonal therapy for breast cancer. There is evidence that weight gain after a diagnosis of breast cancer is associated with an increased risk of recurrence, so excessive weight gain (more than 10 kilograms) should be avoided.

Tamoxifen

Tamoxifen has estrogen-like effects as well as being an anti-estrogen. This means that it acts like an estrogen on some normal tissues but blocks estrogen receptors at the cancer cells. Many women have no side effects with tamoxifen while others report the side effects listed below.

Relatively common side effects include:

- Hot flushes.
- Vaginal discharge: this may be clear or whitish. If it is bloody, you should call your doctor. If it is itchy or has an odor, see your doctor.
- Phlebitis or thrombosis (or both): this is an inflamed vein that contains a blood clot. They occur in about 1% of women taking tamoxifen for 5 years. If the clot dislodges and travels to other parts of the body, particularly the lung, it can be dangerous. Clots are more common in women who have had a previous clot, who smoke, who are inactive, who are getting chemotherapy at the same time, and who have a family history of clots. If you have a swollen or painful leg or calf, see your doctor. If a diagnosis of a blood clot is made, you may need to be on medications to dissolve the

clot and tamoxifen should be stopped.

- Continuation of menses: this is common with premenopausal women. As ovulation can continue, birth control precautions should be maintained as tamoxifen could be harmful to a fetus.
- Endometrial (uterus) cancer: at the recommended dose of tamoxifen of 20 mg given for 5 years, approximately two women per 1000 will develop an endometrial cancer each year. This is two to three times higher than the risk for women not taking tamoxifen. However, for women with an invasive breast cancer more than 1 cm in diameter, the chance of developing endometrial cancer while taking tamoxifen is much less than the benefit of avoiding a breast cancer recurrence. If you have any unexplained vaginal bleeding while taking tamoxifen, you should see your doctor.

Relatively rare side effects include:
- Nausea/vomiting/loss of appetite: usually temporary
- Muscles and joint aches and pains: may be related to menopause
- Rash/skin dryness and hair loss
- Headache, depression, dizziness, decreased memory
- Facial hair: usually subtle
- Fatigue and malaise
- Retinal changes: vision changes have been rarely reported. If you notice a change in your vision, you should get your eyes checked by an eye doctor
- High calcium: occurs rarely when a woman is started on tamoxifen for bone metastases
- Flare up of pain: if there are metastases, these may initially get more painful

Other anti-estrogens

Faslodex (fulvesant) is a newer anti-estrogen that is used in recurrent breast cancer. It is given as an injection every 28 days. It has only been studied in postmenopausal women. Side effects include:
- Nausea and vomiting
- Constipation, diarrhea, and abdominal pain
- Headache

- Back pain
- Hot flushes
- Pain and swelling where the needle was injected

Raloxifene (Evista) is a drug that is very similar to tamoxifen. There are ongoing studies to see if it is a good drug for breast cancer prevention, but the results of the studies are not yet known. It is not presently used in the treatment of breast cancer.

There are a number of other drugs in the same family as tamoxifen that have been studied but are not used or licensed as standard therapy.

Aromatase inhibitors

These drugs are only effective in postmenopausal women as they block an enzyme called *aromatase* that is the last step in the production of estrogen in postmenopausal women. There are three aromatase inhibitors that are used in both adjuvant therapy and in recurrent disease. These drugs are anastrozole (Arimidex), letrozole (Femara), and exemestane (Aromasin). They are very similar in activity and in side effects, and at this time it is not clear if there is one drug that will be shown to be more effective than another.

All these drugs decrease estrogen levels so the most common side effects are those associated with menopause. These include hot flushes, vaginal dryness, and an increased risk of osteoporosis. This last side effect is the most serious and should be part of the discussion about the risks and benefits of taking treatment, particularly in women with very low risk breast cancers.

Relatively common side effects include:
- Muscle and joint aches and pains: these may be mild or more severe and often occur after a woman has been taking an aromatase inhibitor for a while. If they are troublesome, an anti-inflammatory pill such as ibuprofen may be helpful. If they are severe, discuss it with your doctor.
- Increase in lipid and triglyceride levels are seen. These may be of no concern but if you have other risk factors for heart disease such as high blood pressure, a family history, or if you are overweight, you should discuss this with your doctor and possibly take a lipid-lowering drug.
- Loss of sex drive: this could be due to a number of causes, including the psychological stresses associated with cancer,

but it may be worse while taking these drugs.

Relatively rare side effects include:
- Nausea: this usually is temporary
- Headaches
- Swelling of hands, feet, or lower legs if your body retains fluid
- Fatigue and tiredness
- Thinning of the hair is not common but can occur and is usually only mild. If it does occur, it will grow back when you stop taking the drug
- Skin rash
- Depression
- Weight gain
- Vaginal bleeding or discharge
- Diarrhea
- Trouble sleeping

Inhibitors of the pituitary hormones

Inhibitors of the pituitary hormones (LHRH agonists) are drugs that are sometimes used in premenopausal women to put the woman into a temporary menopause by stopping the production of estrogen from the ovaries. This is done by blocking release of the hormones from the pituitary gland that control the ovaries. Studies on a number of these drugs have shown that they are very similar in both their effectiveness and their side effects. Sometimes a combination of an LHRH agonist and tamoxifen is given in addition to chemotherapy or instead of chemotherapy. There are ongoing studies trying to determine the best way to use these drugs and which premenopausal women benefit. These studies are also looking at the combination of an LHRH agonist and an aromatase inhibitor in premenopausal women.

LHRH agonists include goserelin (Zoladex), buserelin (Suprefact), triptorelin (Trelstar), and leuprolide (Lupron). These drugs are all given by a subcutaneous injection and are given on a monthly schedule. Some of the drugs have a long acting formulation (a depot) and can be given once every 3 months.

Side effects include the menopausal symptoms described above. However, studies have suggested that if there is bone loss, it is not permanent and after the LHRH agonist is stopped and ovarian function returns, the calcium content of the bones (the bone density) can return to normal.

Other side effects are rare but may include:

- Pain, tenderness, or redness where the needle was placed
- Increased bone pain during the first 1 to 2 weeks
- Nausea
- Breast swelling or soreness (or both)
- A decrease in sex drive
- Unexpected vaginal bleeding
- Appetite or bowel changes
- Tiredness, headache, depression, dizziness, irritability
- Difficulty in sleeping
- Numbness or tingling of feet and hands
- Swelling of hands, feet, or lower legs if you retain fluid
- Itchy skin rash
- Bone or joint pain
- Changes in eyesight

Other hormonal agents

There are a number of other hormone drugs that are occasionally used in recurrent breast cancer. These include:

Progestins

Megesterol acetate (Megace) is now used infrequently. It is not clear how this drug works, even though progestins have been used in the treatment of breast cancer for many years. Megace is usually well tolerated but there are some side effects and these may include:

- Significant weight gain in 20 to 30% of women.
- Vaginal bleeding
- High blood pressure, headaches, and depression
- Increased risk of blood clots
- Fluid retention, shortness of breath, increased respiratory rate
- High blood sugar levels
- Nausea and vomiting

Androgens

Androgens are male hormones that can be used to treat recurrent breast cancer. The side effects often depend on the dose, how long the treatment is continued, and the individual. Side effects include:

- Masculinizing effects such as scalp hair loss, growth of facial and body hair, lowering of the voice, increase in size of the clitoris
- Weight gain
- Increased sex drive
- Nausea and decreased appetite

SECTION ELEVEN

Chemotherapy

CHAPTER TWENTY-NINE

Chemotherapy: What is it?

CHEMOTHERAPY IS THE USE OF ANY DRUG or medication to treat disease. For example, antibiotics are a type of chemotherapy. Today, however, the word *chemotherapy* has come to refer specifically to the cell-killing (cytotoxic) drugs that are used to treat cancer. There are dozens of different chemotherapy (anti-cancer) drugs. Because they work in different ways, it is common for several drugs to be given at once (combination therapy).

The advantage of chemotherapy and other drug therapies such as hormones (see Chapter 27) is that the drugs travel through the blood stream, reaching cancer cells that may be in distant organs. Drug therapies are therefore also called *systemic treatments* because they attack the cancer through the blood system. In contrast, surgery and radiation are local or regional treatments because the target is one part of the body.

Chemotherapy is used in three ways to treat breast cancer:
- As adjuvant treatment in early cancer to prevent recurrence
- As the main or primary treatment for advanced (high-risk) cancers
- To relieve symptoms and possibly improve survival from cancer that has spread to other parts of the body (metastatic cancer)

Chemotherapy as adjuvant treatment

Many patients with early breast cancer receive chemotherapy after their surgery if their pathology report (see Chapter 12) indicates that there is a risk of the cancer recurring in other parts of the body that may be reduced by giving chemotherapy. Chemotherapy added to the surgery (and often radiation and hormone therapy) reduces the chance of recurrence from cancer cells that cannot be detected but are presumed to still be in the body. The concept of adjuvant (preventive) therapy is discussed more completely in Chapter 22.

Chemotherapy as initial treatment for advanced (high-risk) cancer

Chemotherapy is sometimes used before surgery. The delivery of chemotherapy (or hormone therapy) prior to surgery is called *neo-adjuvant* therapy. Neoadjuvant therapy is used if the cancer is too bulky to be removed cleanly at surgery and sometimes in smaller but aggressive tumours when it is clear that chemotherapy is going to be required. Studies have shown that chemotherapy can be given either before or after surgery to improve survival and decrease recurrence. Neoadjuvant and adjuvant chemotherapy are equally effective.

Larger tumours that cannot be removed cleanly at surgery are called *locally advanced cancer* and are defined as: a) a breast tumour larger than 5 cm in diameter and not easily removed by surgery; b) a tumour fixed (tethered firmly) to the chest wall muscles, the rib cage, or growing into the skin; or c) a tumour of any size associated with large, suspicious-feeling lymph nodes in the armpit.

Usually, a locally advanced cancer is treated with a combination of chemotherapy and radiation instead of or before surgery. Sometimes hormone therapy (see Chapter 27) is used rather than chemotherapy. Once the cancer has become smaller, surgery can be performed to decrease the chance of the cancer recurring in the breast. Inflammatory breast cancer (see Chapter 14) is usually treated in this way as well.

Chemotherapy for treating metastatic cancer

If the breast cancer has already spread from the breast, chemotherapy may be used to slow its growth, to decrease symptoms that

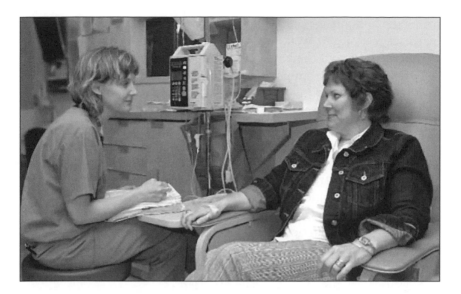

Figure 23: Getting ready for chemotherapy.

are caused by the cancer, to improve the patient's quality of life, and to prolong her survival. A detailed discussion of the treatment of metastatic cancer, including the use of chemotherapy, is included in Chapter 39.

How long does chemotherapy take?

Adjuvant or neoadjuvant chemotherapy is usually prescribed for a 3- to 6-month period. The drugs are usually given intravenously (Figure 23) on one day followed by a 14- to 21-day drug-free rest period and then repeated. Some chemotherapy programs use a combination of oral and intravenous drugs. The alternating treatment and rest periods allow for the maximum cancer-killing effect of the drugs while permitting the body's blood cell counts to return to normal levels during the rest periods (see Chapter 31 on side effects of chemotherapy).

"But I've heard 'horror stories' about chemotherapy!"

Chemotherapy has a bad name due to side effects and fear. Many of the severe side effects people used to experience are no longer a problem. New drugs and schedules have been developed that may be easier to take. As well, drugs have been developed to specifically counteract some of the worst side effects of chemotherapy.

Fear also stems from patients not having a clear idea of *why* chemotherapy is being given. If chemotherapy is recommended as a part of your treatment, it is important for you to fully understand the reasons for it and to ask the following questions:

- Why is the oncologist suggesting it?
- What are the goals of the chemotherapy treatment program?
- How many treatments are being recommended and long will the treatment take?
- What chemotherapy drugs are being prescribed?
- Why is this particular chemotherapy combination being recommended?
- What do I do if I have side effects?
- What are the expected side effects?
- Who should I call if I have problems?

Once you understand the reasons behind the oncologist's choice of chemotherapy and you know what to expect, it is easier to accept some side effects knowing that the treatment is the best possible choice for your particular situation.

Mathematical models to predict risk and benefit

A number of mathematical models have been developed to help health care professionals more accurately assess a woman's risk of recurrence. As well a number of new pathology tests have been developed that are trying to estimate the benefit from chemotherapy for the individual person. These can also be helpful in the discussion between the health care professional and the woman as they may provide an easy to understand graph showing an estimate of both the risk of recurrence with and without treatment as a way of graphically demonstrating the potential benefit of adjuvant drug treatment. One frequently used mathematical model may be found at www.adjuvantonline.com. The model produces estimates of the chance of recurrence if the patient is treated with surgery alone or is treated also with hormonal therapy, chemotherapy, or both. The estimates are based on the best available current data but are just that, estimates. The chance of recurrence predictions from the model are very dependent on accurate information being entered about the pathology and extent of the cancer at the time of diagnosis. As such, the model should only be used as an aid to, and not replace, the consultation with your oncologist.

CHAPTER THIRTY

Who benefits from chemotherapy?

CHEMOTHERAPY MAY BE GIVEN in addition to surgery and radiation when there is a fairly high risk of the cancer recurring. Chemotherapy is not given to everyone because there are side effects. There must be a winning balance between the chance of benefit and the risk of side effects.

The chance of cancer recurrence varies with many factors, some of which we understand and some of which we don't. Table 7 describes how patients may be grouped into broad categories of low, medium, and high risk and the sort of adjuvant treatment that would be justified based on this risk grouping. New information is continuously coming available that helps make these estimates more accurate.

Like all treatments, taking chemotherapy is not a guarantee that the cancer will not come back. Studies are trying to determine who will benefit from chemotherapy and which chemotherapies will be most useful. Ask your oncologist to give you an estimate of your benefit of receiving chemotherapy. This is often most understandable as the number of women per 100 treated in your situation who will be alive 10 years later because they had the chemotherapy. It is less helpful if the estimate of benefit is described as a percentage reduction (for example 30%) in the chance of recurrence.

As well, since there is no reliable way of knowing exactly which women have been cured by surgery alone and which women will be cured by chemotherapy, recommendations are made based on your tumour's characteristics. There is no current test that can reliably tell us if you, individually, will benefit.

Table 7 General basis for recommendations for adjuvant hormonal and chemotherapy		
Lowest risk (10% or lower risk of recurrence after 10 years without therapy)	**Moderate risk** (10 to 20% risk of recurrence after 10 years without therapy)	**High risk** (greater than 20% risk of recurrence after 10 years without therapy)
All of: Tumour less than 1 cm *plus* no cancer in nodes *plus* no invasion into lymphatic or blood vessels of the breast *plus* estrogen receptor positive, and HER2 negative **Treatment:** No adjuvant chemotherapy; may consider hormonal treatment or no drug treatment	**All of:** Tumour less than 2 cm *plus* Grade 1 or 2 *plus* no cancer in nodes or invasion into lymphatic or blood vessels of the breast and estrogen receptor positive Tumour less than 1 cm and estrogen negative or HER2 positive **Treatment:** Hormone treatment if ER or PR positive Chemotherapy if ER negative Chemotherapy and anti HER2 therapy if HER2 positive	**Any one of:** Tumour larger than 2 cm diameter Tumour larger than 1 cm *plus* Grade 3 or HER2 positive or triple negative Tumour with nodes that contain cancer and/or invasion of lymphatic or blood vessels in the breast **Treatment:** Hormone therapy if ER or PR positive and discussion about chemotherapy Chemotherapy if triple negative Chemotherapy and anti-HER2 therapy if HER2 positive (and hormone therapy if also ER/PR positive)

Recommendations for adjuvant (postoperative) chemotherapy

Adjuvant chemotherapy may be recommended if one or more of the following situations is present:

- A tumour is estrogen, progesterone, *and* HER2 negative (called a *triple-negative* tumour) that is 1 cm or larger. Triple-negative tumours smaller than 1 cm may be considered high risk as well.
- A tumour is HER2 overexpressing. HER2 overexpressing tumours less than 1 cm may not have a recommendation for chemotherapy, especially if less than 5 mm.
- A tumour is high grade (Grade 3), especially if it is estrogen and progesterone receptor negative or HER2 positive and greater than 1 cm diameter. Tumours with a Ki67 score of more than 13% may also be considered high risk even if not Grade 3.
- Cancer cells have spread to the lymph nodes or have invaded the lymphatic or vascular channels of the breast.
- A woman is 35 years old or younger even without other risk factors.
- An Oncotype DX Recurrence Score of greater than 31. This is a commercially available test that has shown a benefit for chemotherapy in hormone positive patients with scores above 31. The benefit of chemotherapy in hormone-sensitive tumours with recurrence scores in the range of 18 to 31 is being tested and currently needs to reviewed on an individual basis.
- An ER+ tumour greater than 5 cm in diameter even if there are no other high-risk features.

Chemotherapy is more likely to be recommended if tumours are estrogen receptor-negative, as they do not respond to hormonal therapy. Chemotherapy is also more frequently recommended for HER2 overexpressing tumours (HER2 positive) as they are known to have a higher risk of recurrence than a similar HER2 negative cancer, and anti-HER2 therapy is most effective when given together with chemotherapy.

The decision to use chemotherapy depends upon the extent of the cancer, the tumour's estrogen receptors, the HER2 status, the other options available for therapy, and the woman's age (younger women may have a higher risk of recurrence) and the general state of the woman's health. Considering all these factors, women may be offered chemotherapy if their cancer has a moderate or high risk of recurrence (see Table 7).

Why is chemotherapy recommended for these women?

Chemotherapy is recommended when there is a reasonable likelihood that the benefits—avoiding cancer recurrence—outweigh the risk of side effects. The estimate of benefit is based on knowledge of the properties of the cancer as discussed in Chapter 12. The most important factors in determining if a cancer will recur and how well it will respond to chemotherapy are the size of the cancer, whether it involved lymph nodes at the time of diagnosis, the grade of the cancer, the estrogen receptor content, and the HER2 status.

When hormone therapy is less likely to work

Tumours that are not sensitive to estrogen or progesterone will not respond to hormone therapy and therefore chemotherapy is the only systemic therapy with proven benefit at this time. If the cancer has a moderate or high risk of recurring (Table 7) and does not have estrogen or progesterone receptors, chemotherapy will usually be recommended.

Grade of the cancer

Studies have shown that cancers that look aggressive under the microscope (Grade 3, Chapter 12) tend to recur more frequently. Women with Grade 3 cancers that are greater than 1 cm in size may benefit from chemotherapy, even if they are sensitive to hormones.

HER2 status

Women with tumours that have too much HER2 (overexpression) have an increased risk of recurrence and may be offered chemotherapy even if there are no other high-risk features. Herceptin, an anti-HER2 antibody, is useful if the woman's tumour overexpresses HER2. Other anti-HER2 treatments may become available in the future.

Age

Women younger than 35 years of age often have a more aggressive cancer. Chemotherapy and hormonal therapies may be recommended just because of a young age.

Cancer-involved lymph nodes

Cancerous lymph nodes in the axilla (armpit) indicate a moderate or high risk of cancer recurrence. Surgery alone will cure only a minority of these women because the cancer cells have often escaped outside the breast before surgery.

If the tumour is sensitive to hormones and has a low or moderate grade, chemotherapy may not be recommended. However, if there are several involved nodes or if the cancer is Grade 3 or HER2 positive, chemotherapy is usually recommended.

Cancer invading the lymphatics and veins of the breast

If the pathologist sees cancer cells in the lymphatic channels or veins of the breast, there is a higher risk that the cancer has spread beyond the breast. As with women with involved lymph nodes, adjuvant chemotherapy may be recommended if the pathology report describes cancer cells in these areas.

A large cancer

The size of the cancer is very important. A 1-cm cancer is made up of about one billion cells. The larger the cancer, the higher the risk that some of these cancer cells will have escaped and be growing outside the breast. Some lower grade cancers that are very large may have a risk of recurrence that is high enough to recommend chemotherapy.

What's best for you

As the understanding of breast cancer improves there will be changes in the recommended treatment. As well, treatment policies may vary somewhat in different centres. Apart from these changes, what is most important is for you to understand why chemotherapy has or hasn't been chosen for your particular case and for you to feel confident that the best possible choice of treatment has been made.

CHAPTER THIRTY-ONE

Side effects of chemotherapy

Why are there side effects?

ALL DRUGS, EVEN ANTIBIOTICS or headache tablets, have side effects. What counts is that the beneficial effects of a drug outweigh the problems or discomforts of its side effects. Knowing that a particular drug or combination of drugs can effectively destroy the cancer, you may be more willing to tolerate the side effects, especially if they're temporary.

It is important to be aware of possible side effects before beginning treatment and to discuss them with your doctor. This will make the chemotherapy process less mysterious and frightening and allow you to decide for yourself whether the benefits warrant the side effects. Knowledge of side effects also makes you an active participant in your care. You can help self-manage some side effects and be more confident when it is time to ask for help, even on weekends and holidays.

Although a number of side effects are predictable, others are not. For example, some chemotherapy drugs always cause hair loss while other drugs rarely affect the hair. Different people can also have different reactions to the same drug. In the last few years a number of drugs have become available that have decreased the most feared side effects—nausea and vomiting.

Drug names and drug combinations

An important point to note about drug names is that all drugs have two names: a chemical or generic name, and a brand name. For example, headache tablets have brand names such as Aspirin and Tylenol, but the chemical name for Aspirin is acetylsalicylic acid and that for Tylenol is acetaminophen. When you are discussing a particular drug with your doctor, ask him or her to tell you both the chemical name and the brand name (write them down). Since the two names are often used interchangeably, being aware of both will help you avoid confusion.

Different chemotherapy drugs work in different ways. To take maximum advantage of this, the drugs are often given in combinations—attacking on all fronts. Because certain combinations are used frequently, you may see them referred to as abbreviations. Some typical examples used in persons without HER2 overexpression are:

- AC: Adriamycin and cyclophosphamide
- AC-Taxol and dose dense AC-Taxol: Adriamycin, cyclophosphamide and paclitaxel (plus or minus G-CSF)
- CAF (or FAC): cyclophosphamide, Adriamycin and 5-FU
- CMF: cyclophosphamide, methotrexate, and 5-FU
- DC: Taxotere and cyclophosphamide
- FEC (or CEF): cyclophosphamide, epirubicin, and 5-FU
- FEC/DOC: cyclophosphamide, epirubicin, and 5-FU and docetaxel
- TAC or AC-Docetaxel (Taxotere, Adriamycin, cyclophosphamide)

All of the above drug names are chemical (generic) names except for the brand names Adriamycin (its chemical name is doxorubicin), Taxotere (chemical name is docetaxel) and Taxol (the chemical name is paclitaxel).

When the tumour is HER2 positive, a drug named trastuzumab (Herceptin) is commonly given with or after the chemotherapy. Other anti-HER2 drugs are being developed and tested in research studies and may be approved for use in the near future. Some of the chemotherapy protocols used in HER2 positive cancers are:

- AC-Taxol/Herceptin and dose dense AC-Taxol /Herceptin: Adriamycin, cyclophosphamide paclitaxel (plus or minus G-CSF) and Herceptin

- FEC/DOC and Herceptin: cyclophosphamide, epirubicin, 5-FU, docetaxel and Herceptin
- TCH: taxotere, carboplatin, and Herceptin

Any of the other regimens may also be given with Herceptin following the treatment but are less commonly used.

The side effects

Hair loss

Losing your hair is often the most difficult part of chemotherapy. Some chemotherapy drugs such as doxorubicin, epirubicin, paclitaxel, and docetaxel cause baldness in everyone if given at a high enough dose although at lower doses they may not. Other drugs such as cyclophosphamide (Cytoxan) cause more variable hair loss from thinning or total baldness, and others such as 5-FU cause almost no hair loss at all.

Hair loss occurs because the chemotherapy slows down the rapidly dividing cells of the roots of the hair. Thinning usually begins about 2 weeks after the first dose of chemotherapy. You will notice that you are shedding in the shower, on your brush, and on your pillow. The hair breaks at or near the skin, so the scalp may be tender. The chemotherapy may also cause thinning of the hair on the rest of your body, including your eyebrows, eyelashes, arms, legs, and pubic hair. The hair grows back, sometimes even during the chemotherapy, and it is usually already a few inches long by the third month after finishing the drugs.

Hair loss is the most upsetting event for both women and men as it is a public symbol of your cancer. In most situations it cannot be avoided, but fortunately it is temporary. Buy a wig before it happens and take it to your hairdresser to get it styled so you are prepared. If you have long hair, a couple of gradual haircuts could make the change less startling for yourself and your family. Hats, turbans, and scarves can be very helpful.

Although there have been attempts to decrease hair loss by scalp hypothermia (cold packs on the scalp) or electrical stimulation of the scalp, these are generally uncomfortable and variably effective. Furthermore, because the cold decreases blood flow to the area, many doctors are concerned that the amount of chemotherapy delivered to that area would be reduced, possibly leaving a potential cancer site untreated.

Infection

White blood cells in the blood stream protect the body from infection. Many chemotherapy drugs reduce the white blood cell count and this often occurs about a week after the injection. If the white blood cell count drops too much or stays down too long, your body's defense mechanisms are low and you have a higher risk of getting an infection. Severe infections can be life-threatening.

How can you protect yourself? You don't need to become a hermit but you should take precautions:

- Wash your hands frequently, especially after using the toilet and before cooking, eating, or handling any food
- Take good care of your skin by taking frequent showers or baths
- Use a soft toothbrush
- Use an electric shaver rather than a razor
- Report painful conditions in the anal area
- Be on the alert for any signs of an infection

If you get a fever, sweats, chills, a cough with yellow or green phlegm, burning urine, a sore that will not heal, diarrhea, or any other signs of an infection you should call your doctor or the on-call doctor immediately so antibiotics can be prescribed. It is rare to require hospitalization, but oral antibiotics may be needed for about 5 to 7 days until your white blood cells recover.

The white cell count usually recovers about 21 days after chemotherapy, which is why many courses of chemotherapy are given in sessions separated by 3-week breaks from chemotherapy. If your white cell count hasn't recovered enough to make it safe to give another dose of chemotherapy according to the schedule, then treatment will be delayed or the doses will be reduced.

A hormone called *granulocyte colony stimulating factor* (G-CSF, Neupogen, Neulasta Filgrastim, Pentagastrin) may be prescribed if you have problems with infection, a very low white blood cell count, or if you are prescribed frequent doses (for example, every 2 weeks) of chemotherapy. The G-CSF is a synthetic form of a natural hormone that helps your bone marrow recover and increases your white blood cell count after it has been lowered with chemotherapy. G-CSF is given as an injection under the skin (subcutaneously), similar to an insulin injection, either by the patient or a nurse every day or sometimes every other day for 3 to 14 days. Pentagastrin

(Neulasta) is a long-acting formulation and can be given once every 2 or 3 weeks.

Do I need to stay home or avoid crowds during chemotherapy?

It is important for you to live as normal a life as you can during chemotherapy so you do not need to stay home for the entire time. But use common sense. If you do not need to go into a hospital to visit someone, don't go. If you know someone has a bad pneumonia or cold, stay away. Avoid unnecessary exposure but you do not need to stay home all the time.

What happens if my husband, partner, or children come home with a cold or infection?

Again, use common sense. Use frequent and complete hand washing techniques, avoid too much physical contact (kissing) during the infectious time, and watch for any signs that you may be getting ill, such as developing a fever.

Anemia

The number of red blood cells in the blood stream may also be reduced by chemotherapy, but it does not usually drop too much.

Anemia may cause you to feel tired, dizzy, short of breath, or chilly, so if you notice any of these symptoms you should report them to your doctor. Although you should eat well, anemia caused by chemotherapy is not usually helped by taking iron or B vitamins since the low red blood cell count is not caused by nutritional deficiencies but by a decreased production of red cells. If your anemia becomes severe enough to cause symptoms, (often when the hemoglobin falls to less than 100 g/L) your doctor may recommend a blood transfusion.

Abnormal bleeding or bruising

Platelets help to clot the blood. Chemotherapy may cause a temporary decrease of the platelet count. If this is severe enough, you may bleed easily. It is rare for low platelet counts to be a significant problem, but if you notice any abnormal bleeding or bruising you should report it to your doctor. ASA (Aspirin) or ibuprofen (Advil) drugs can slow down platelet function and may be taken but you should confirm you are using these medications with your chemotherapy doctor. Acetaminophen (Tylenol) does not affect the platelets and is generally okay to take in moderation.

Nausea and vomiting

Many of the chemotherapy drugs cause nausea and vomiting, although some people are affected more than others. Antiemetic drugs, which prevent nausea and vomiting, are usually given before the chemotherapy and every few hours afterwards for the first 24 to 48 hours. The nausea may start 6 to 8 hours after the chemotherapy injection, or even the next day, and is usually not a prolonged problem. Eat something before the chemotherapy and regularly thereafter because it is often better not to have an empty stomach.

The nausea may feel like morning sickness, so it is sometimes helpful to take an antiemetic, have something to eat (for instance some dry crackers) and stay in bed for an hour to prevent vomiting. Avoid odors that cause more nausea. If the drugs you are given to prevent or treat nausea are not effective, tell your doctor so that different or additional antiemetics can be tried.

The drugs used to prevent nausea and vomiting include ondansetron (Zofran), prochlorperazine (Stemetil), dimenhydrinate (Gravol), metoclopramide (Maxeran), nabilone (Cesamet), and dexamethasone (Decadron). Other drugs such as Emend may be used in conjunction with some of the drugs listed above if the nausea is very severe. Diphenhydramine (Benadryl) and lorazepam (Ativan) may also be helpful. Note that these drugs may also have their own side effects. For example, ondansetron (Zofran) may cause headaches and constipation and prochlorperazine (Stemetil) may cause restlessness that could require yet another drug, diphenhydramine (Benadryl), for relief. The drugs may be given as pills, intravenous or intramuscular injections, or as rectal suppositories. The suppositories may be very helpful if you are vomiting or nauseated.

Some people also complain about stomach pain, an acidy feeling, heartburn, and a change in the taste in their mouth. These symptoms may be eased by food or antacids, but if the symptoms are severe, particularly the pain, you should notify your doctor. Some persons find taking a regular medication to decrease the acidity of their stomachs such as ranitidine (Zantac) or rabeprazole, for the months of chemotherapy is helpful.

Diarrhea and constipation

The anti-cancer drugs often cause some change in your bowel habits so don't be alarmed by minor disruptions. If you have severe diarrhea for more than 24 hours, or cramps, you should call your doctor because an anti-diarrheal drug may stop the problem. As well, you should be assessed to make sure this was actually related to the chemotherapy and not something totally unrelated. A stool culture may be necessary to ensure that you do not have an infection. If you have diarrhea, try to drink lots of clear liquids to replace the fluid that you have lost and to rest your bowels. Avoid foods such as cabbage, beans, brans, and spicy foods that cause loose bowels, gas, and cramps. Milk products may also contribute to diarrhea.

Some chemotherapy drugs and some of the antiemetics may cause constipation. Often this can be avoided by drinking plenty of fluids, keeping active, and possibly taking a mild stool softener. If you have a severe problem, notify your doctor.

Sore mouth (mucositis)

Many of the chemotherapy drugs cause soreness or dryness of the mouth and throat that can appear about 5 days after treatment begins. If this is a problem, avoid foods that irritate your mouth such as acidic, spicy, or rough foods. Rinse your mouth often with baking soda and water. If your mouth gets so sore that you cannot eat, notify your doctor, as there are special mouthwashes and painkillers that may ease your discomfort. People who tend to get cold sores (herpes) in addition to other mouth sores can be helped by an antiviral medication. If a white, cakey covering develops in your mouth you may have a yeast infection (candida), which can cause mouth soreness and difficulty eating and swallowing. An anti-fungal mouthwash or pill may help.

Menstrual periods and sexuality

Chemotherapy may disrupt your menstrual periods, causing them to be irregular, to stop temporarily during chemotherapy and then return, or to stop permanently. This is not predictable, but it is more likely to happen in women closer to menopause than in younger women or if you are taking 6 months of chemotherapy rather than 3 months (see Menopause, below). If you are having menstrual changes, discuss them with your oncologist.

Chemotherapy drugs generally do not affect the ability to have sex, although you may notice changes. The mucosal lining of the vagina may feel dry or sore. Lubricating gels such as Replens, Muko,

Astroglide, or Slippery Stuff may be helpful. As well, chemotherapy may increase the risk of getting a vaginal yeast (candida) infection, which may irritate the area and may require treatment with anti-fungal creams. Certain sexual positions could cause discomfort to your arm or chest area after surgery. Your libido, or sexual desire, may be affected by the stress of the illness, fatigue, your anxiety, and the changes in your body that may affect your hormones, self-confidence, and your body image. These are natural and normal responses that may be temporary. If you have continued difficulties with your sexual interest or activity, you and possibly your partner may want to discuss strategies to rekindle your sexuality with a professional counsellor. Most cancer centres have persons specialized in sexuality on staff or to whom you can be referred.

Menopause

Menopause is simply when menstrual periods stop completely, and is usually defined as 1 year without periods. We now know that the hormonal changes that occur with menopause normally develop over a decade or so. At menopause the ovaries stop releasing eggs and stop making estrogen. This decrease in the level of estrogen causes changes in the body in a wide variety of organs and tissues. In some women these changes are subtle and do not cause any problems. In other women they are troublesome and cause upsetting and frustrating symptoms.

Chemotherapy can bring on an early and abrupt menopause in some women due to the effect of the drugs on the ovaries. This is more common in women over the age of 40 and may depend on which drugs are used and the total doses prescribed. In some women the periods stop temporarily; in others they stop permanently. Even with blood tests and symptoms, it is sometimes difficult to know how complete the menopause is for a few years as some women have a return of their periods quite a time after they stopped.

Menopause is a natural occurrence for all women but the symptoms of menopause are often a distressing part of the cancer treatment, particularly as it may come earlier and more abruptly than a natural menopause. Menopause can be associated with the following symptoms and changes:
- Hot flushes/flashes
- Dryness of the vagina and perineum
- Dry skin

- Weight gain
- Mood changes
- Increased risk of osteoporosis (thin bones, decrease in the calcium content of the bones, and increased risk of bone fractures). Bone loss is called *osteopenia* when it is mild and *osteoporosis* when more severe
- Increased risk of heart disease
- Memory changes
- Changes in libido (interest in sex)

Menopause is not the same for all women. It is important to have a discussion with your doctor about the symptoms. If women in your family have a significant history of developing heart disease or osteoporosis at a young age, there may be specific precautions that you should start early if you become menopausal. Your doctor may want to assess your bones with a bone density test even if you do not have a family history. This test is like a bone scan but shows whether there is evidence of osteopenia or osteoporosis.

To avoid some of the problems associated with menopause:

- Stop smoking. It can cause heart disease, osteoporosis, lung disease, and cancer.
- Exercise regularly. Weight-bearing exercise can protect against osteoporosis; aerobic exercise is important for your heart and weight. Exercise may be helpful in avoiding recurrence.
- Check your diet. Ensure that you have 1500 to 2000 mg of calcium in your diet or as supplements, 1000 to 2000 IU of vitamin D, and a low-fat diet that is not too high in calories.
- For vaginal dryness: a water-soluble lubricating jelly (e.g., Replens) can help maintain vaginal fluids. Lubricating gels such as Replens, Muko, Astroglide, or Slippery Stuff can also make intercourse less painful. Occasionally, estrogen creams may be used sparingly. Estring is an intravaginal low-dose estrogen.
- If you have hot flushes, try to reduce your stress and limit your intake of caffeine, alcohol, chocolate, and cola, as they can worsen hot flushes. Some women have some relief with evening primrose oil, Remifemin (black cohosh) or other herbal remedies. Prescription drugs that may help include Effexor, Dixarit, Bellagral, or Neurontin (gabapentin). The use of estrogens and progesterones (Megace or DepoProvera)

for women with a history of breast cancer remains controversial, but these medications are being studied to assess their safety. If used they should be used sparingly after a discussion with your doctor about other options.

- Osteoporosis may be treated with medications such as biphosphonates (etidronate, clodrinate, Fosamax), which decrease the bone changes, and occasionally with progesterones and estrogens. New agents such as denosumab may be effective. Raloxifene (Evista) is a medication similar to tamoxifen and licensed for the treatment of osteoporosis. It may be helpful but is not a substitute for tamoxifen and there are concerns about long-term (more than 5 years) use.
- For changes in libido: It may just take time to get used to your body's changes. Occasionally, testosterone is recommended, as it may help encourage your sexual interest. Because testosterone can be converted into estrogen in your body, its use after a diagnosis of breast cancer is controversial, especially if the tumour was ER-positive.

It is important to remember that there is not one solution for all women. Menopausal changes and concerns are highly variable.

Prevent pregnancy during chemotherapy, but not with "the pill"

Taking chemotherapy does not necessarily prevent pregnancy. Furthermore, *it is important not to get pregnant while on chemotherapy* because these drugs, especially during the first 3 months of pregnancy, may cause damage and deformity of the fetus. While on chemotherapy, it is important to continue to use birth control measures; these should be discussed with your doctor. As your periods could be irregular, it may be difficult to predict the time of ovulation, so a combination of a barrier method (a condom or diaphragm) plus a spermicidal foam or gel is safest. Oral contraceptives are generally *not* recommended if you have breast cancer because estrogens may stimulate the growth of some cancers.

Fertility after chemotherapy

Many women ask about having a baby after they have finished chemotherapy. If you continue to have periods and ovulate you may be able to get pregnant, but you should wait until you are fully recovered from the treatment and until you and your oncologist have discussed the risk of the cancer coming back. Pregnancy itself will not cause the cancer to come back, but the unpredictable nature of breast cancer and its potential for recurrence needs to be considered prior to a pregnancy.

If you are pregnant when you are diagnosed with breast cancer, chemotherapy may be given if you are in your second or third trimester and if it is important to begin treatment right away.

Increasingly women want to ensure they can have a child after chemotherapy and are storing eggs or embryos. This requires a lot of coordination as there is the need for ovarian stimulation and harvesting before the chemotherapy starts, and often takes a month or 6 weeks. In some situations there is not time to wait but in other situations, particularly if the woman sees the fertility expert as soon as the core biopsy confirms cancer, it can be facilitated. There may be concerns about the hormones used for the ovarian stimulation but there is no evidence that a short course of ovarian stimulation causes an increased risk of cancer spread.

There are some reports that using an injection to stop periods (goserilin, brand name Zoladex, or buserelin, brand name Suprefact; see Chapter 28) prior to and during chemotherapy may protect the ovaries from being damaged and becoming permanently menopausal. There are also techniques in which a part of the ovary is removed. Fertility should be discussed as soon as the cancer is diagnosed, and a consultation with a fertility expert or clinic could be arranged. Delaying chemotherapy for 4 to 8 weeks to complete the fertility assessment and preservation procedures is usually acceptable.

General symptoms

All chemotherapy drugs may cause skin changes such as dryness, spots, increased sun sensitivity, or rashes. If you are going out in the sun, wear protective clothing, including a sun hat. Many women complain about dry, gritty eyes, which can be eased by eye drops or artificial tears. Other women complain of a flu-like feeling or of feeling cold for 1 to 3 days after the chemotherapy starts.

If the drug contains a dye (for example Adriamycin, which is red) your urine may change colour the day after you start chemotherapy as you excrete the drug. You do not need to take special precautions in the bathroom, as the chemotherapy drugs are not dangerous to anyone else. You should drink plenty of fluids to ensure a good urine flow and to prevent bladder irritation.

Some women develop joint or muscle aches and pains. These often begin after the chemotherapy is finished and can last several months. Fortunately, they are usually temporary and can be relieved with exercise or anti-inflammatory medications.

Certain drugs may cause tingling in the fingers and toes, and some people report a loss of muscle strength and a change in their sense of balance. This also should be temporary. If it is not, or if it interferes with your activities, report it to your doctor.

Some women complain of "chemo brain," a loss in their short-term memory. This is often temporary. Studies have confirmed that some memory loss may occur during or shortly after treatment. It is difficult to know if the memory loss is due to the chemotherapy, the stress of the illness, the cancer itself, or all the anti-nausea and other medications that are taken. It is also not known if there are any long-term effects (more than 2 years) or how many women are significantly affected.

If you experience any new problem, report it to your doctor. It may or may not be related to the chemotherapy. If you have finished your treatments and are on follow-up, you should probably report it to your family doctor, since the issue may be unrelated to the therapy.

Other considerations while taking chemotherapy

While you are on chemotherapy, you can eat whatever you like. However, if you are taking medication for another condition, your doctor should verify that it can be continued. Although some physicians and nutritionists recommend total abstinence from alcohol, an occasional glass of wine or beer is usually okay.

Fatigue levels vary. Some women are able to continue their normal activities and continue working throughout chemotherapy. Others find chemotherapy so physically or emotionally draining they need to take a prolonged leave from work. Although it is recommended that you remain as active as you can while on chemotherapy, you will need some extra rest. It is hard to predict how much rest you will need. It is advisable to sit down with your family or your employer and warn them that there will be low-energy days.

Physical activity is important. If you exercise regularly you might want to continue, but tone down your routine to avoid straining yourself. For example, walks may replace your daily jogs. Many centres have exercise programs or recommendations.

PART THREE | **Beyond
the initial phase
of treatment**

Coping with cancer

Living with a diagnosis of breast cancer: Tips for you, your family, and your friends

EVERY PERSON WITH CANCER and every family member is unique, but the road each must travel is well worn by the millions of others who have come before. It is a journey marked by hope and despair, courage and fear, humour, anger, and uncertainty.

There is no "right way" to feel after receiving a cancer diagnosis

Many women are concerned that the thoughts and feelings they experience following a diagnosis of cancer are somehow abnormal or crazy and that there must be a "right way" to feel. This couldn't be further from the truth. There is no one way to feel. Reactions to the diagnosis can span the full range of human emotion: anger, anxiety, uncertainty, hopelessness, helplessness, depression, a feeling of isolation, vulnerability, relief that there really is something wrong, and even guilt that one has somehow contributed to the development of her own disease or delayed in bringing it to a doctor's attention.

It is important to realize that the initial reaction to the diagnosis will be followed by other feelings. Just as we go through a series of stages in accepting the loss of a loved one, we pass through a number of emotional levels on our way to acknowledging the diagnosis of cancer. First, there is often disbelief in the diagnosis, denial that it is true, and anger at the feeling of being singled out. Finally, there is usually an acknowledgement that "Yes, I do have cancer."

Denial is often a prominent response early in the cancer experience. It is a defense against fear and helps to maintain emotional equilibrium. It is not uncommon to hear people comment, "I think she's in denial," as if there may be something unusual and potentially dangerous about this reaction. In fact, some degree of denial is normal and is probably necessary to protect oneself and to maintain the hope needed to participate in daily life. However, it is important to recognize that denial is healthy only as long as it does not interfere with seeking medical care or participating in appropriate treatment.

Expressions of very strong emotion are to be expected and they may range from anger and bitterness to frank hostility that may be directed at anyone and anything.

Fortunately, most people will emerge from the storm of emotions to reach a point of equilibrium and acknowledgement. It is common to move back and forth from one stage to another. Many think about having cancer in the past tense, which helps to keep the cancer from dominating a woman's life and allows her to remain more positive, even if she is well aware of the possibility of recurrence.

Coping with cancer

Every person has a unique tool box of coping strategies that have been accumulated over a lifetime. Most will find what they need to cope with cancer. Seeking information, maintaining hope, turning to family and friends for support, developing a partnership with the health care team, and learning stress management techniques are all ways to develop the coping mindset. Many women take this time as an opportunity to learn new coping strategies from health care professionals and other women who can help them and their families cope with this new experience.

Seeking information

Appropriate information can help to allay much of the anxiety and fear associated with the unknown. The type and amount varies with the needs of the woman and her family. Generally, people want to know about diagnostic tests, the treatment plan (purpose, expected results, side effects, length of time, and scheduling), and prognosis. Essential but often neglected information includes how the disease and treatment are likely to affect the person's daily life and work. Your cancer centre and support groups provide this kind of help. There are booklets, seminars, stress management training programs, and self-help groups for individuals with cancer and their families.

Of course, the health care team is a critical provider of information pertinent to your particular problem. When attending appointments, ask questions. Prepare a list; otherwise, you may forget important points that you have been wondering about. Write down the answers and, ideally, take someone along to help you remember what was said. Have your accompanying person take notes for you so that you can concentrate on the consultation. One can be in a daze during the early phase of diagnosis and treatment, so having an extra person to listen, take notes, and clearly recall is very helpful. Another strategy is to audio-tape the consultation with your oncologist(s). Ask permission to do this in advance; most oncologists are comfortable with this practice.

Telling others

In most cases, your family and close friends will learn sooner or later that you have cancer. It is usually best to disclose the information yourself, according to your own schedule. Confiding fears and hopes is an important part of developing the coping mindset and, in the long run, it is easier than trying to conceal these important feelings.

Telling young children that their mother has cancer can be especially painful. A woman usually feels tremendous anxiety about how best to inform and explain to children when she is trying to cope herself. Most women are worried about being able to care for their children during treatment and about whether they will be around to help them grow up. The goal in telling children is to give them opportunities to ask questions about the disease and to express their feelings about it. While we all wish to shield our children from bad news, it is better that they experience pain in a way that they understand and can talk about with their parents. Coping with sorrow on their own in forms that become embellished by their imagination is far less reassuring than open discussion with their family. Moreover, if children are not told what is happening, they may become confused and hurt and mistakenly believe that they are responsible. They may also imagine things that are not true. They need to hear what is happening in real language from their parents to be reassured that they are included and respected. There are several excellent books available which can help you explain cancer to children of various ages (see Additional Reading). Also, there may be support groups for children at your cancer centre.

Support groups

In most cities and towns there are support groups consisting of people with cancer and trained professionals or volunteers who manage the sessions. The session leader provides a forum where the person with cancer can be open about her thoughts and feelings, and can discover that these are normal and acceptable. Other members of the group often suggest alternative ways to deal with difficult issues, ways that have helped them. Seeing others who are coping with similar situations can help you identify solutions to problems that initially seem overwhelming. In addition, membership in a formal group may help you overcome a feeling of helplessness because you will be offering assistance to others. Support groups can also provide information. As the group participants learn about their disease they may approach problems and find solutions in different ways. Many women find sharing their experiences with others to be helpful. Increasingly, online, virtual support groups are being shown to be effective ways for people to create communities of common interest, including cancer support groups.

A word of caution about support groups

Participating in a support group requires an investment in time and energy that may compete with family or other activities. You may experience unexpected emotions in some group sessions. For example, you could be upset by the beliefs or coping mechanisms of other group members. Some groups may not be led by appropriate individuals with reliable skills or information, and unintended emotional consequences could result. If you feel uncomfortable or something does not feel right about any particular group, it is best to leave immediately and seek another group.

Reach to Recovery Program

The Reach to Recovery Program is a one-on-one support system managed by the Cancer Society. It can be a valuable resource for women with a new diagnosis of breast cancer. The Reach to Recovery volunteers have all had breast cancer themselves. The program tries to match women for direct contact either in person or by telephone.

Information about the Reach to Recovery Program or to make a referral can be done through the Cancer Information Service. In Canada, this service is at 1-888-939-3333.

Developing a partnership with the health care team

At one time, patients and families were considered to be silent members of the health care team, if indeed they were considered members at all. Today, people with cancer are encouraged to take an active role in treatment planning.

Find out who the players are

The first step in developing a partnership with the health care team is to know who the players are and what each one has to offer. This can be a challenging task as, over time, there are often many different specialists involved in the care of the patient and family. Try to identify one team member who will serve as the leader or navigator: often the family doctor, the oncologist (cancer specialist), or a specialist nurse. It doesn't matter who assumes the role as long as he or she is able to relate to you and your family and will be there for the duration. This person should be available at regular intervals, or when required, to listen to concerns, to direct questions to the appropriate professionals, and to act as a guide and support.

Participate in decision making about treatment

No matter how complex your problem may seem, your health care team members should be able to help you participate in the decision-making process by providing you with understandable information and the framework of the big picture. Start by taking the time to be informed and make treatment choices about the first decisions in front of you. Then get more informed about subsequent steps in the treatment journey and participate actively in the various treatment choices that present themselves. The educational process continues through the cancer journey.

Participating in decision-making involves listening to the options, identifying their advantages and disadvantages, and comparing them with your family's and especially your own values and aspirations. Some women want to discuss all of the options, perhaps seeking a second opinion before making an informed decision with or without their families. Others might be uncomfortable making the final decision, but can still participate by clarifying their values and wishes so that the final recommendations for treatment are tailored to their needs. Ask questions so that you make an informed decision with which you are comfortable.

Participate in treatment planning

Participation in the treatment planning includes managing the side effects of the treatment, reporting changes in condition, attending follow-up appointments, providing team members with feedback about how things are progressing, and using the services and supports that are available.

When friends don't call

Lost and strained friendships can be a particularly painful aspect of dealing with cancer. Friends may not call for a variety of reasons. For most, it is because they feel that they will have so little to say that will help, and they fear that instead they might say something hurtful or disturb you when you want to rest. Others are afraid that they will not be able to respond appropriately to your change of appearance, or they are fearful of facing the possibility of your death and the eventuality of their own.

If you believe it is discomfort that is keeping a particular friend from visiting, you might try a phone call to dissolve the barrier. This often reassures them that you are still the same person that they liked before, and that you understand their difficulty. However, don't expect to change or enlighten everyone. We all have our own emotional capabilities and some people cannot be comforted enough to help them maintain the same relationship. You will find that different friends will provide support in different ways at various times, and you will also make new friends along the way who are participating in the same treatment process.

Sexuality and fertility

Sexuality need not be affected by the diagnosis of breast cancer but it often is. Many women feel damaged by the surgery and uncomfortable with their bodies. Also, treatment can cause fatigue and other symptoms that decrease desire. The onset of treatment-induced menopause may make intercourse uncomfortable due to vaginal dryness. This can be treated.

The whole process of the diagnosis and treatment may make a woman less interested in sex. Her focus may shift to other issues or she might feel depressed. This is normal and needs to be openly discussed with her partner. Her partner may also be frightened about losing or hurting her. A common myth is that cancer could be contagious. This is entirely false.

By recognizing changes and seeking counselling if necessary, these feelings may improve with time and understanding. Be assured that a satisfying sexual relationship is possible after breast cancer but may take time to establish.

Fertility may be a concern for younger women with breast cancer. Chemotherapy can interfere with the function of the ovaries and may cause temporary or permanent infertility. For a more in-depth discussion of fertility and pregnancy issues, see Chapter 40.

Maintaining hope

Hope is a crucial tool for people with cancer and their families. It is an internal resource that permits one to cope with the stresses associated with diagnosis and treatment. Loss of hope reduces one's ability to adjust to the situation.

Hope means different things to different people, and tends to change over time depending on the stage of the disease and treatment.

Maintaining and nurturing hope is a strategy that can allay anxiety, depression, and fear. Nurturing hope means focusing on the present and what is immediately ahead, rather than on the future or the past, neither of which can be changed. While this reorientation of focus can be difficult, it can help you manage the daily challenges of cancer treatment.

Hope can be affected by the behaviour of others. Family members and friends can support the idea that being hopeful is a good thing, and they should not classify hope as being false.

Hope is not based on false optimism or benign reassurance, but is built on the belief that better days or moments can come in spite of the situation.

How can friends and family help you cope with breast cancer?

Practical support

While loved ones may feel powerless to help you with the cancer, they are eager to do something practical or tangible to lighten your load. Practical help is very important during breast cancer treatments and this help comes in many forms. For example, one thoughtful person organized a "meals on wheels" for her friend during her radiation treatment. Another woman vividly recalled how her elderly father got up nightly to feed her 4-month old son so that she could rest longer.

Ask friends or family members to take you to your chemotherapy and radiation treatments and clinic appointments in order to be that extra listener. You could also ask them to bring over your favourite food or to do the grocery shopping or the laundry. Let them clean the house, mow the lawn, and look after the car. They could help with child care. Accept their offers to take you to a humorous movie or play.

You could ask a friend to go wig and hat shopping with you. Or ask for hats as gifts, instead of flowers. Of course, flowers are nice too, as is the occasional box of chocolates! Get your friends to help you with holiday preparations. During treatments, you may be too tired to write Christmas cards or thank-you notes. If you want to send cards and notes, your friends or relatives could help you write them.

Single women living alone report welcoming daily telephone calls from friends and family. These women also sometimes appreciate friends or family spending nights with them, especially when they were feeling particularly ill or vulnerable. A daughter might move home to be with her mother, or a sister might move in during treatment.

Financial stresses may be particularly troublesome for women who work to support themselves or their families. Some of the treatments may need to be paid by the patient herself. The social work or counselling departments of your regional cancer centre should be able to provide useful information and assistance to access benefit programs such as Pharmacare, employment, or disability insurance, or emergency financial aid.

Emotional support

People sometimes appreciate being listened to unconditionally, especially when they need to rant and rave or feel sorry for themselves. We all need someone with whom we can do that. Friends and family members who are not afraid to talk about breast cancer are helpful. If the woman feels her friends or family members are not able to hear these things, she may spend a lot of time reassuring them that she is fine, although she may suffer from being unable to unburden herself.

Many women want to be hugged, especially when the tears are flowing. Some draw strength from frequent phone calls and visits. Many enjoy going for walks with friends. Receiving letters and cards can be welcome and reassuring. Humour is often appreciated.

There may be times when you want privacy and do not wish to speak to anyone. However, your friends and family still want to know how you are faring and how they can help.

It's useful to ask one reliable friend or relative to be an intermediary, to field calls and questions on your behalf. This person need not be your best friend or a family member, but should be someone whom you can trust to pass along information so you don't have to answer the same question about your cancer, again and again. This person can let other people know what you need during treatments and rough times. She or he can also let your network know what would make your life more pleasant and less stressful.

Your intermediary can draw up a list of your needs and wants and ask your friends how each of them can contribute, emphasizing that each participant is to take on only what they can commit to and no more. Support may be needed for the long haul and it's important not to burn out friends and family. Driving children to dance classes, shopping chores, gardening, returning books to the library—the list is endless and unique to each person. Spreadsheets can be very useful in keeping track of who is responsible for doing what. Let your friends adopt the "many hands make light work" approach. Including others as part of your treatment and recovery can be a gift to your helpers as well as yourself.

You may experience mixed feelings about self-help books, motivational tapes, megavitamin diets, or herbal remedies offered with the best of intentions by friends and relatives. Some women appreciate this type of advice and muster the energy to take it to heart. For others, gifts that possibly imply that one is somehow responsible for their disease only make them feel angry or guilty.

Many women resent advice to think positively, wondering if the implication is that if she had been a positive thinker, she would not have breast cancer. Relatives and friends have to bear in mind that it may be difficult to think positively, let alone get out of bed in the morning, when you're exhausted by your treatment.

Vulnerable times

The weekend before your first treatments can be a very anxiety-ridden time for you. That's when it's important for your friends and family to rally round and listen to your fears or help you with practical chores.

You may also have a difficult time when your breast cancer treatments come to an end. Suddenly, you will no longer be under the intense scrutiny of your health care providers and you may feel somewhat abandoned. Your ongoing fears of the cancer returning may escalate at this time, especially as you are no longer occupied with therapy. Your family and friends need to be made aware of these fears so that they can support you. Breast cancer is a frightening disease that can undermine you on every front. However, sympathetic relatives and friends can support you and, as one woman reported, "help you get your life back."

Feeling vulnerable after your treatment is completed

Many women feel anxious or low after completing their treatment and do not know where to turn. Their hair has grown back, they are back at work, their family is happy everything is back to normal, but they are anxious. This is very common and may be because the cancer experience has changed the woman. She may still be living the cancer experience while everyone around her wants to move on. Anxieties about recurrence, the future, and how to cope are common. Also, many women want to maintain some of the things they learned during the experience of treatment but do not know how to do this.

This is a time when it is important to seek counselling or support groups where you can learn how to deal with the anxieties about recurrence and talk to other women who are re-entering a new "normal" phase of living. Take this time as an opportunity to make changes you may want to make and to learn to live a happy life that is not dominated by cancer fear.

CHAPTER THIRTY-THREE

Exercise, physical therapy, and management of lymphedema

EXERCISE HAS BEEN SHOWN to have a beneficial effect on health at any time of your life. Regular aerobic exercise, which increases your heart and breathing rate, can promote a good night's sleep, improve your overall sense of well-being, assist in maintaining ideal body weight, and keep your heart and lungs working effectively. As well there is recent evidence showing that exercise may be beneficial in both preventing the initial development of breast cancer occurrence and reducing the chance of recurrence. Whether this is related to an effect of maintaining a normal body weight (see Chapters 4 and 35) or whether there is a specific mechanism by which exercise works is not clear. Research studies are ongoing looking at the role of exercise in breast cancer treatment.

Many breast cancer treatments such as surgery, radiation, and chemotherapy have side effects that can be reduced or eliminated by physical therapy. Preventing physical limitations can help restore and maintain your overall health and fitness and enhance your quality of life. Exercise medicine experts and physiotherapists may provide individualized care but here is a summary of general exercise principles.

Physical therapy after surgery

Breast cancer surgery requires removing the tumour, from the breast and an inspection of the axilla with often a sentinel node procedure and sometimes a full axillary dissection (see Chapter 19). After any type of surgery, one can expect some pain, discomfort, stiffness, and swelling. This is especially true after axillary dissection. Up to 50% of women who undergo this procedure develop tightness, pain, and the formation of "cords" in the armpit, inner elbow, and wrist within a few weeks after their surgery. These thin, visible cords are the hardened lymphatic vessels that have been interrupted by the removal of axillary lymph nodes. Some reduction in the range of arm motion may occur temporarily due to cording. Usually, within several weeks, the cords will rupture and arm motion will return. An axillary dissection or radiation to the regional lymph nodes may also lead to difficulties in shoulder motion and weakness, and can contribute to lymphedema or arm swelling. Some women require physical therapy to return to their presurgical levels of shoulder motion and upper body strength, especially if they had an axillary dissection.

Aerobic exercise is helpful during and after chemotherapy and radiation therapy

Although chemotherapy and radiation may make you feel tired and it is important to get extra rest, you may feel better if you maintain or improve your overall fitness by exercising 3 to 5 days per week. During treatment you may not be able to do as much exercise a you could do before, but regular activity is important. For maximum benefit, you should exercise at least 3 to 5 days a week, and it is generally recommended that you do 20 to 60 minutes at each session. Activities that involve large muscle groups, such as brisk walking, jogging, swimming, cycling, rowing, or skating have the greatest benefit. If you have not done regular exercise before, start out slowly, but commit yourself to doing it regularly. For example, walk four times around a track at your local high school and time yourself. If you don't like walking on a track, use your car to measure the distance of a pleasant walk through your neighborhood. Or, walking on a treadmill in a community centre allows you to time your walking speed and measure the distance walked. Continue to walk 1.5 kilometres (1 mile), three to five times a week, but try to gradually increase your speed over several weeks. It is more important to get into a regular habit of walking than to increase your speed. When you can walk 1.5 kilometres (1 mile) in 15 or 16 minutes, increase your distance to 2 kilometres (1.5 miles).

What about exercise after chemotherapy treatment?

Chemotherapy can also cause joint pain or stiffness similar to arthritis-like pains. Regular exercise that is gentle on your joints, such as walking or swimming or riding a stationary bicycle, may help during this period. Moist heat such as hot packs or a warm bath can help ease joint and muscle aches. Also, cold packs can help reduce acute (sudden) joint pain or swelling.

After menopause women lose the protective benefit of estrogens for the bones. Chemotherapy and hormonal therapies may further affect the bones and increase the risk of osteoporosis. Strengthening and weight-bearing exercises counteract the bone loss of osteoporosis and are therefore particularly important. A physical therapist or an exercise specialist can suggest a conditioning program for you.

Exercises to regain the range of shoulder motion after surgery

An important problem to tackle after surgery is to regain full shoulder motion. Some women regain full motion within days after their surgery, but many women have trouble. This is seen especially when trying to: a) lift your arm forward in front of your face (shoulder flexion), b) raise your arm out and up at the side (shoulder abduction), and c) bring your arm behind your back to fasten a bra (shoulder internal rotation). The following exercises can help you regain these motions. The exercises should be started gently when the drain, if any, is removed. This will usually be within the first week after surgery. Exercise may progress to more active stretching by the second week. Doing these exercises will not break anything, nor will they harm the healing process following surgery.

The first two exercises should be done while lying on your back on the floor. In the first exercise (Figure 24), use a broomstick or cane to have the uninvolved arm help stretch the involved arm into the full range of shoulder flexion. Stretch slowly, as far as you can comfortably go, exerting a prolonged pull on the affected arm. In the second floor exercise (Figure 25), put your hands underneath your head and slowly bring both elbows down to the floor. Breathe out as you stretch and try to get your elbows to touch the floor. Then relax and breathe in. Breathe out again as you try to stretch a bit further. Repeat each of these exercises four to five times, making sure that your stretches are slow, steady, and prolonged.

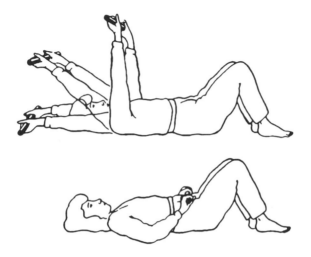

Figure 24: Holding a broomstick helps the unaffected arm stretch the affected arm in this exercise. (Figures 24 to 30 used with permission from *Recovering from breast surgery: exercises to strengthen your body and relieve pain*. Diane Stumm, Hunter House, 1995.)

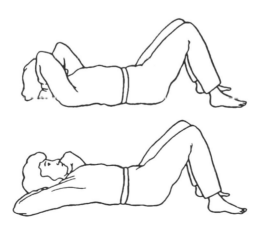

Figure 25: With hands behind your head, elbows are slowly brought down to the floor.

The third shoulder stretching exercise (Figure 26A) is performed while sitting in a chair or on the floor. It helps to do this exercise in front of a mirror. Once again, use a slow, steady, and prolonged stretch to pull your affected arm up over your head and toward your ear. After each stretch, lower your arms and relax. Repeat the stretch four to five times. Once you can do this comfortably, you can increase the pull by bending your trunk sideways toward the side opposite to the involved arm (Figure 26B).

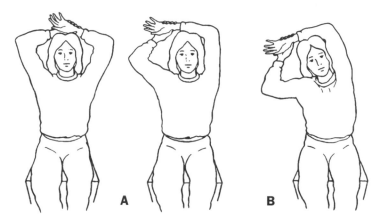

Figure 26: The affected arm is slowly and steadily stretched over your head.

The next two exercises will improve shoulder flexion. Stand facing a wall, with your feet about 15 cm (6 inches) away from the wall (Figure 27). Try to walk the fingers of both hands up the wall while standing in place. When you have gone as high as you can comfortably go (while feeling a slow, prolonged stretch to your underarm muscles), hold that position for 5 to 10 seconds to maintain the stretch. To gauge your progress, put a pencil mark at the furthest point to which you can walk your affected arm.

Another shoulder flexion stretch (Figure 28) is done while you are on your hands and knees on the floor. With your hands directly underneath your shoulders and with your knees about 25 to 30 cm (10 to 12 inches) apart, slowly lean back on your feet and lower your head to the floor. Keep your elbows straight and feel the pull in your underarm area. Hold the stretch for 5 to 10 seconds and then return to the hands-and-knees position. Repeat the stretch four to five times.

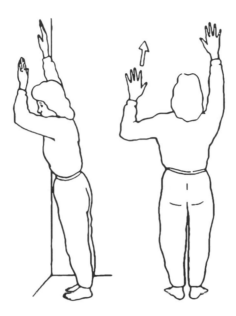

Figure 27: Walk your fingers slowly up the wall, and then the stretch for a few seconds.

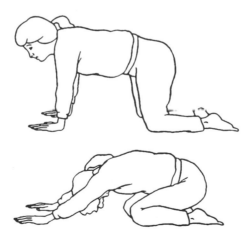

Figure 28: Slowly lean back on your feet and, with elbows straight, lower your head to the floor.

Strengthening exercises

It used to be said that vigorous exercises should not be done after breast and axillary surgery. This is no longer true. Once you have full shoulder range of motion, at 4 to 8 weeks after surgery, you can begin to add exercises to increase upper body strength. In the stretching exercise shown in Figure 24, for example, you can add a 1 to 2 lb. (½ to 1 kg) weight in each hand and alternately stretch each arm up over your shoulder to strengthen the shoulder muscles. To create your own 1 lb. weight, fill a small plastic detergent bottle with sand or pebbles. Or, you can hang a weighted bean bag (2 to 3 lbs.) over the broom handle or cane and use this to assist in strengthening.

Because the chest muscles are often weakened, especially if you have had a mastectomy, you can strengthen these muscles by doing push-ups while standing against a wall (Figure 29) or from a hands-and-knees position (Figure 30). For the standing push-up, stand with your feet about half a metre) (about 2 feet) apart. Place your hands on the wall, slightly outstretched, at the level of your head. Lean forward to touch your forehead against the wall. Push away slowly until your arms are fully extended. Repeat 8 to 12 times. To make the exercise harder, move your feet back further away from the wall.

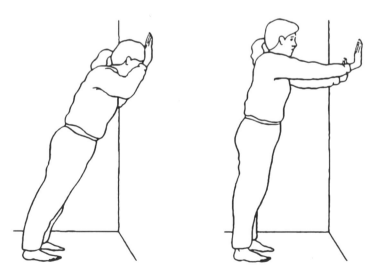

Figure 29: With feet away from the wall, bend your elbows and bring your forehead to the wall. Remember to keep your back straight.

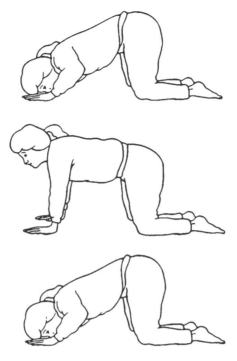

Figure 30: With knees slightly apart and hands wider than your shoulders, do a push-up, lowering your head until it touches the floor.

The second type of push-up is from a hands-and-knees position (Figure 30). With your knees slightly apart and your hands placed slightly wider than your shoulders, lower your head until your nose touches the floor. Then, straighten your elbows until your arms are fully extended. Repeat 8 to 12 times.

If you had an axillary dissection

Because your lymphatic system has been interrupted as a result of the axillary dissection, it may be advisable to wear a compression sleeve on your affected arm when doing weight-training involving more than 10 to 15 lbs. (or any other strenuous upper body exercises). This is especially true if using weight-lifting equipment. When using weight machines such as a bench press or latissimus pull-down, start with the smallest weight possible and increase very gradually. The greatest benefit is derived from weight-training if it is done at least twice a week with a minimum of 8 to 12 repetitions of each exercise.

Lymphedema

Women who have had axillary dissection can develop lymph-edema (swelling) in the affected arm. Lymphedema occurs because the lymph fluid, which bathes the tissues in your arm, can no longer leave the arm through the lymphatic channels in your armpit. Between 5 and 20% of women who have had an axillary dissection will develop permanent lymphedema, usually within 2 years after their treatment. The risk is much lower in women who had a sentinel node biopsy without axillary dissection. Most of the time the lymphedema is minor but sometimes it can be severe. Some women (5 to 10%) develop temporary lymphedema, which disappears within a few months after breast cancer treatment.

To determine if lymphedema is present, the circumference of both arms needs to be measured. It is recommended that measurements be made using a tape measure at four specific points on your arm: at the mid-palm of the hand, wrist, 10 cm below and 15 cm above the elbow. Any measurement that is 2 cm greater on the affected side than the non-operated side is considered to be significant lymphedema.

Treating lymphedema

If you develop lymphedema you will need help from a physician, physical therapist, nurse, massage therapist, and, if the condition of your arm is causing you to be depressed, a psychosocial counsellor.

For temporary lymphedema, elevation of the arm, a compression sleeve worn with activity, or close monitoring may be all that is required. Permanent lymphedema may require compression therapy, which involves the use of a compression sleeve or pump. Compression pump therapy can be carried out several times a week or as needed. Physical therapists specializing in lymphedema care offer pump therapy and compression garments, as do many cancer centres.

A form of massage to stimulate lymphatic drainage, called *manual lymph drainage* (MLD) or *manual lymph treatment* (MLT), is gaining popularity. It involves bandaging and special exercises and is usually carried out by massage therapists. Complex physical therapy (CPT) or complex decongestive therapy (CDP) is a treatment program which combines MLD, bandaging, exercises, support garments, and skin care counselling to control lymphedema.

Lymphedema is easier to control if you are not overweight and if you exercise regularly. It used to be said that if you have lymphedema you shouldn't do active exercise with your arm, such as playing tennis, squash, lifting weights, rowing, or cross-country skiing. Recent studies do not support these precautions and suggest, instead, that exercise is far more beneficial than harmful. Your arm will certainly let you know which activities worsen the lymphedema. You may want to wear a compression sleeve during vigorous upper-body exercise.

Avoid scratches, burns, cuts, and bruises to your involved arm. When you need procedures to be done, such as having blood drawn, intravenous lines started, or injections given, try to have them done on your healthy arm. Also, injuries can cause swelling or infection that is not handled well by the stagnant lymphatic system in your affected arm. Therefore, always be on the lookout for signs of infection in your arm (painful redness of your skin) and get immediate treatment. The infections are almost always caused by bacteria called *streptococci*, which respond well to penicillin. You should have some antibiotics on hand to be taken at the first sign of infections, especially if you are travelling to a remote area.

Preventing lymphedema

The following are key points for helping to prevent problems from lymphedema if you have had an axillary dissection:
- Try to maintain an ideal body weight because obesity is a risk factor for lymphedema.
- Try to avoid having your blood pressure taken, blood drawn, injections or vaccinations, or intravenous lines started in the involved arm. If you have had bilateral mastectomies, use the arm that did not have lymph nodes removed. If both sides had lymph nodes removed from the armpit, alternate which arm is used.
- Protect your arm from cuts, scratches, and infections by wearing an oven mitt rather than using a pot-holder around the stove and oven. Also wear a gardening glove and long sleeves while digging, pruning, planting, or berry picking.

- Consider wearing a compression sleeve when lifting heavy weights or engaging in vigorous upper-body exercise such as cross-country skiing, rowing, or tennis. It used to be thought that you shouldn't do active exercise, but that advice has changed in recent years.
- Report any signs of arm swelling, pain, or redness or any suggestion of infection to your health-care provider immediately.
- Consider wearing a compression sleeve when you fly, particularly on a long flight. There is no compelling evidence to show this is of benefit but if you have had problems with arm swelling after an airplane flight it may be worthwhile considering.

CHAPTER THIRTY-FOUR

Reconstructive surgery

Should I or shouldn't I?

NOT ALL WOMEN ARE INTERESTED in breast reconstruction. Some feel that the cancer operation itself is quite enough. Others will opt for additional surgery to reconstruct the breast. It is a personal decision and no particular way is right. The most common reason for breast reconstruction is the psychological desire to feel whole again. The goal is to restore self-image and self-confidence and improve quality of life.

Women seeking breast reconstruction need to be physically and mentally healthy, must understand the associated risks and complications, and be motivated from within. They should not be undertaking reconstruction to please others in their lives. Occasionally, a patient's poor health or poor prognosis from their disease means that they cannot be considered for this operation. Also, some women are emotionally unprepared to undergo further surgery, with its related risks and potential complications.

Breast cancer treatment always takes precedence

Breast reconstruction should not interfere with the treatment of the patient's breast cancer. The breast cancer surgeon, plastic surgeon, and oncologist should ensure that the plans for reconstruction

SECTION TWELVE – COPING WITH CANCER

are integrated into the cancer treatment program. Reconstruction generally does not interfere with detection of possible recurrence of the cancer on the chest or elsewhere in the body.

The first visit to the plastic surgeon

Your breast surgeon, family physician, or oncologist usually arranges the initial referral to a plastic surgeon. During your first visit, the plastic surgeon will ask you questions about your expectations, desires, and general health, and do a brief physical examination. The plastic surgeon will discuss the available reconstructive options and explain your preferred option in greater detail. You should ask questions about the options available, details of the surgical procedure, the degree of pain, the recovery time, and the risks. Expect the surgeon to provide diagrams and photographs or introductions to other patients so that you acquire a realistic sense of the possible results and what to expect during the postoperative recovery period. While every surgeon has produced excellent results, breast reconstruction is not an exact science and possible postoperative complications and patient factors may contribute to a result that falls somewhat short of your expectations.

Factors that affect the choice of reconstructive procedure

Reconstruction is designed to correct surgical changes. The type of procedure recommended will depend on the type and extent of the surgery (see Chapter 19), but other factors also influence the choice of procedure and the expected cosmetic result. These will differ from one woman to another and include the amount and looseness of the skin, direction and length of the original surgical scar, the amount of fat under the skin, the possibility of skin changes caused by radiotherapy, and the shape and size of the other breast. An additional factor relates to the timing of the reconstructive surgery. Reconstruction surgery can be done at the time of mastectomy (immediate reconstruction) or at some time following recovery (delayed reconstruction). The choice of method will depend on the combination of your wishes, the surgeon's and oncologist's preference, the type and extent of the cancer operation, and the nature of the opposite breast.

Surgical techniques: Implants or Tissue reconstruction

Implant reconstruction

A tissue expander is a device that looks like an empty plastic bag with an attached valve. It is surgically placed behind the pectoralis muscle. In the weeks following surgery, the expander is inflated using a small amount of saline (salt water). The idea is that after the surgical site has healed, the bag can be enlarged gradually by injecting salt water into the valve every 1 to 2 weeks. Like the abdominal skin during pregnancy, the skin of the chest will stretch as the pseudo-breast enlarges. Usually, this process goes on for several months in order to overstretch the skin to a size larger than the normal breast. Then, a second operation is done to

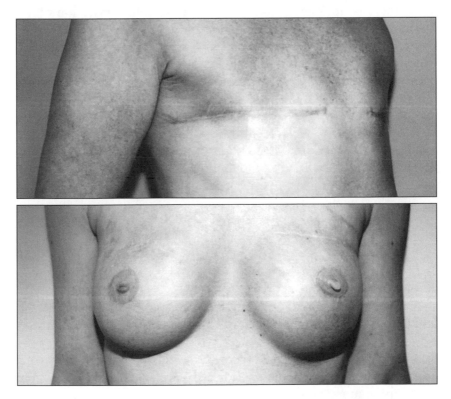

Figure 31: The result of breast and nipple reconstruction of both breasts. Tissue expanders were used to stretch the skin from the preoperative stage (upper) until there was sufficient room for the implants to be inserted. At a later operation the nipples were reconstructed (lower).

remove the expander and replace it with a permanent breast implant (Figure 31).

An implant is a fluid or silicone-filled bag shaped like a small round or oval cushion. The implant is typically placed through a portion of the old incision, against the ribs, tucked underneath the pectoralis muscle. The surgery is done under general anaesthetic and usually involves a brief hospitalization. Postoperatively, there may be drains in place to remove any fluid build-up, and there will often be more pain than from the original mastectomy.

Most often, reconstruction involves a two-step procedure: insertion of the tissue expander and later, removal of the expander and insertion of the implant. Occasionally there is enough skin and normal tissue remaining after the mastectomy that an implant can be inserted directly. The use of a tissue expander is appropriate when there is not enough skin remaining to allow insertion of an implant large enough to match the volume or shape of the other breast. Many surgeons who use tissue expanders believe that by overstretching the skin, there will be a more natural droop to the breast after placement of the permanent implant.

Complications of implant reconstruction include infection, bleeding, or problems related to the implant itself, such as the development of a layer of scar tissue around the implant. This scar tissue forms a fibrous capsule around the implant that may contract and squeeze the implant into a firm, round ball. This is called *capsular contracture*. If this happens the implant will feel firm and will retract up the chest wall. This may be unsightly and uncomfortable and may require more surgery to correct it. The chance of developing capsular contracture in the absence of previous radiation is approximately 10 to 20%. However, when radiation is used before or after an implant-type reconstruction, approximately 50% of patients will develop capsular contracture.

The most common disadvantage of the tissue expander-implant form of reconstruction is failure to achieve a shape similar to the opposite breast. Another disadvantage is that it involves two operations (as do most breast reconstructions) and extra visits to a doctor's office for the fluid injections. In addition, saline (salt water filled) implants may leak and deflate. If this occurs, more surgery will be required to replace the implant with a new one. This type of reconstruction is not generally used if there has been radiation to the breast or chest wall skin.

A newer method of implant reconstruction is a one-stage procedure using a permanent silicone filled implant that is placed partially behind the pectoralis major muscle, which acts as a protective cover for the upper half of the implant. The lower portion is protected by a cover of treated, sterilized, recycled human skin. This cover does not have any living cells and provides a frame for the body's fibrous cells to grow into. This framework provides protection and decreases the formation of a hard capsule around the implant. It is not available everywhere and there are ongoing studies to evaluate the results and cost of this method.

Over the past decade, textured saline implants and tissue expanders have been introduced in the hope of decreasing the risk of capsular contracture and optimizing the shape of the reconstructed breast. However, there is a tendency for these devices to become relatively immobile on the chest wall and patient satisfaction with the textured saline implants has been low except in patients in whom reconstruction of both breasts is required.

Tissue-based reconstruction

Tissue reconstruction techniques involve shifting a piece of your own tissue that includes skin, fat, and often muscle from one part of the body to another. The tissue that is shifted or transferred is called a flap. Often, a portion of the flap remains attached to its original site to ensure that the tissue in the flap has an adequate blood supply. Other times the flap is attached to blood vessels in the new area using microvascular surgical techniques that connect the veins and arteries to each other using an operating microscope. The rationale for the use of these tissue flaps is that by using the body's own tissue, a more natural-feeling breast may be created, avoiding the complications related to implants. However, there is a trade-off. Tissue reconstruction is more complex surgery and involves increased risks, scarring, potential donor site problems, and longer recovery time.

A myocutaneous flap includes muscle and skin

In one type of myocutaneous flap operation, the latissimus dorsi muscle (the large triangular muscle from the back) along with the overlying skin is moved into the mastectomy area. For some women, enough tissue can be transferred from the back to create a good breast size (medium B cup). If a larger breast is required, this pro-

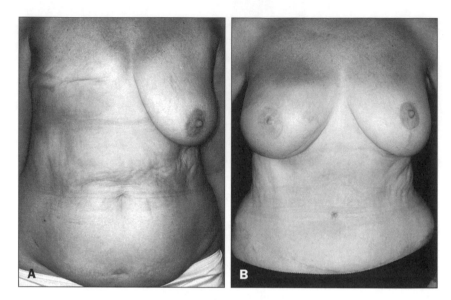

Figure 32: Preoperative (32A) and one year postoperative (32B) appearance of a woman with a delayed transverse rectus abdominus muscle flap reconstruction and left reduction mammoplasty carried out for symmetry. The abdominal scar is just visible above the panty line. At a second operation the right-sided nipple was created.

cedure can be combined with a small implant to optimize volume. However, this operation leaves a scar and a contour deformity on the back and eliminates the latissimus as a functioning muscle in the back (Figure 32). Surprisingly, most women are not aware of this lost function afterwards. The hospital stay is approximately 2 to 3 days. Often, the woman is discharged with a drain in the back donor site and will require home care until the drain is removed.

Probably, the most commonly used flap technique is the transverse rectus abdominus muscle flap, known as the TRAM flap. This type of surgery will usually produce the best results for patients who are highly motivated, have a suitable abdomen, and are willing to tolerate a longer recovery phase. This method uses a large section of skin and fat from the lower abdomen (belly) along with a portion of one of the rectus (sit-up) muscles, which provides the blood supply to the tissue. A breast mound is fashioned out of the skin and fat that has been brought up from the abdomen (Figure 33).

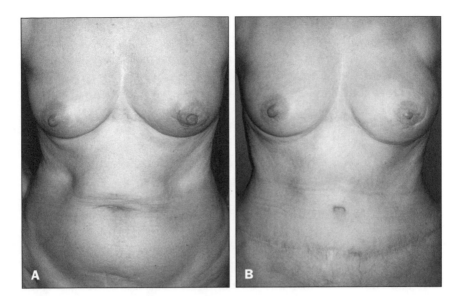

Figure 33: Preoperative (33A) and one year postoperative (33B) comparison of a woman who had an immediate TRAM flap reconstruction of the left breast. A skin-sparing mastectomy was done through the small circular scar surrounding the left areola in 33B, and the patient's own nipple and areola was removed along with the underlying breast tissue. The breast mound is composed of tissue transferred from the site of the new abdominal scar. In a second-stage operation, the nipple and areola in 33B were fashioned surgically and with tattooing.

The abdominal defect from where the muscle is taken (donor site) is repaired with sutures, and sometimes requires reinforcement with surgical mesh. Postoperatively, the woman is mobilized slowly and typically spends 4 days in hospital. The abdominal area is more uncomfortable than the chest as a result of muscle spasms. Drains will be present at the breast site as well as in the abdomen donor site, and will gradually be removed as the amount of drainage decreases. Recovery time is usually 6 to 12 weeks, depending on the patient. Strenuous abdominal activity is discouraged for 6 to 8 weeks. The amount of time off work averages 6 to 12 weeks; however, some patients require more time.

Although using the body's own tissue sounds attractive, this is a complex method of breast reconstruction, with additional possible complications, including abdominal wall hernia (2 to 5%), part of the flap not surviving (5 to 20% in nonsmokers, higher in smokers), thrombophlebitis (formation of blood clots in the veins), healing problems in the abdominal site, and postoperative lung problems (rare). If reconstruction is done at the time of mastectomy, there is an increased risk of a portion of the mastectomy flap not surviving in about 10 to 15% of patients. Although this may not ultimately affect the overall reconstructive result, it requires extra wound care and dressings to the area over a period of several weeks.

Women at highest risk for complications are those with large, heavy breasts, diabetics, smokers, those with chronic lung disease, immune arthritic conditions, or those who have had previous radiation therapy to the breast or chest wall. The reason for the added risk is that these conditions affect the adequacy of blood flow into the flap. Good blood flow into the flap is essential to proper healing and function of the flap tissue. These patients should only be considered candidates for flap surgery if the surgeon has extensive experience in these techniques and the patient is extremely motivated and understanding of the potential risks. Most surgeons require patients to quit smoking beforehand, ideally 2 to 3 months prior to TRAM flap surgery. Another issue that may prevent the use of a TRAM flap is the presence of other surgical scars in the abdomen that may have disrupted the necessary blood supply to the abdominal tissue.

A side benefit of TRAM flap breast reconstruction is a free tummy tuck (Figure 32). However, if a patient has had a previous tummy tuck procedure, they can no longer be considered for this surgery. Previous abdominal liposuction can also increase the risks associated with the TRAM flap procedure, and may have reduced the available fatty tissue to an inadequate volume for this type of operation.

Second-stage breast reconstruction

Most breast reconstruction should be viewed as a two-stage surgical procedure. The first step is to create a new breast mound using one of the techniques already discussed. Creation of the breast mound itself may require two operations if a tissue expander followed by permanent implant method is chosen. The second stage occurs 4 to 6 months later to optimize symmetry between the two breasts and to reconstruct a nipple. This is usually a minor procedure compared to the creation of the breast mound. If the original reconstruction was a flap procedure, then minor scar revisions may be done at this time.

Nipple reconstruction

Many women who seek breast reconstruction are happy once a breast mound has been created. Other women will opt to also have a new nipple and areola reconstructed. Typically, a projecting nipple can be made from small flaps of tissue raised up locally off the previously created breast mound (Figure 32), or it can be taken from the opposite nipple as a graft if the opposite nipple is large. The more darkly pigmented areola can be fashioned from a portion of the opposite areola or a skin graft from high on the inside of the thigh, or it can simply be tattooed. Nipple-areola reconstruction is relatively minor surgery. The main problems relate to partial graft failure, loss of projection of the reconstructed nipple, and mismatched colour. The new nipple will not have any sensation.

Matching the breast exactly

Paradoxically, the easiest situation to achieve identical-looking breasts (symmetry) is when both breasts are reconstructed (Figure 31). When only one breast has had surgery, the goal of reconstruction is to create a new breast shape that as closely as possible matches the normal breast, but an exact match is seldom possible. To get a close match, the normal breast may need to be altered. This may require a breast uplift (mastopexy) or reduction of the normal breast. Both of these procedures create some scars on the normal breast, and introduce some risks and potential complications. Despite this, symmetry surgery of the opposite breast is generally very well tolerated and often gives the patient a more youthful, less heavy and droopy breast that more closely matches the reconstructed breast (Figure 32).

Timing of breast reconstruction

Traditionally, breast reconstruction after mastectomy was delayed for a period of time, often a year, to allow time to complete additional therapies such as radiation and chemotherapy, and to allow the woman to recover mentally and physically from her ordeal before she proceeded with more extensive surgery. Alternatively, the reconstruction procedure may be done at the same time as the mastectomy. Advantages of this include reducing the number of operations and reducing the necessary recovery time and time off work, lessening the body image disturbance and grief reaction that many patients suffer after mastectomy, and optimizing the overall cosmetic result by allowing a skin-sparing (skin-saving) mastectomy (Figure 33). However, despite the improved cosmetic results that are often attainable with immediate reconstruction, patients in this group are often less satisfied with their reconstruction result compared to those who have had to live with a mastectomy deformity for a period of time prior to reconstruction.

Disadvantages of immediate reconstruction include the coordination of two surgeons, a longer operation, and a potentially increased number of complications. Some oncologists prefer that if additional therapies such as chemotherapy and radiation are going to be necessary and the patient is at high risk for wound healing complications (smokers, diabetics, obese patients, large-breasted patients), that reconstruction be done as a delayed rather than immediate procedure. Timing of reconstruction, then, is a decision that should be made in consultation with the patient, the oncologic surgeon, and an oncologist involved in the patient's care.

Timing of radiation with reconstruction

Even with a mastectomy and reconstruction there may be a need for radiation therapy, especially if the tumour was large or involved the lymph nodes. The presence of a tissue flap or implant does not affect the ability to deliver radiation therapy or the effectiveness of the treatment. However, there are additional factors to consider, including the time to heal from the reconstruction surgery, the need for chemotherapy, and that the use of radiation therapy increases the risk of complications such as fibrosis and capsular contracture if an implant type of procedure is used. Especially if a mastectomy and immediate reconstruction is contemplated, preoperative consultation with the surgical, reconstructive, radiation oncology, and medical oncology teams should be done. The intended use of radiation may influence the type of surgery the plastic surgeon will recommend. In addition, if the preoperative status of the tumour indicates that radiation therapy is highly likely, this may be done as part of a neo-adjuvant program with the mastectomy and reconstruction done as the final phase of treatment rather than the first phase.

SECTION THIRTEEN

Lifestyle issues

CHAPTER THIRTY-FIVE

Nutrition

WE EAT TO SATISFY a complex set of needs—emotional, cultural, sensual, and of course, nutritional. Eating well, in every sense of the word, is one of the most important things that a woman with breast cancer can do for herself.

Is there a link between diet and breast cancer?

Among other factors, diet may influence the risk of developing breast cancer. However, the importance of diet in comparison to other more established risk factors such as reproductive and genetic factors is unknown. Certainly many women who eat healthy can, and do, develop breast cancer.

Nevertheless, the consumption of alcohol increases the risk of breast cancer. In addition, being overweight and weight gain in adulthood may raise the risk of developing breast cancer in postmenopausal women. Diets high in fat may increase the risk of developing breast cancer but the evidence is less clear. A large Canadian study did not find that a low-fat diet reduced the chance of developing breast cancer. Other lifestyle factors such as regular exercise may lower the risk of developing breast cancer.

For more information see Canadian Cancer Society's guide-book *Eat Well, Be Active: What you can do* (2009) or visit www.cancer.ca.

The benefits of a good diet after diagnosis of breast cancer

Recent research findings show that factors such as diet, exercise, and maintaining a healthy body weight likely play a role in breast cancer recurrence and survival. Aside from cancer treatment, lifestyle choices may have the greatest impact on reducing the risk of recurrence and improving overall health. Eating a plant-based diet that is rich in vitamins, minerals, fibre, and protective compounds, as well as foods low in fat may reduce the risk of breast cancer recurrence. Achieving and maintaining a healthy body weight is also important, and this is more easily achieved on a lower calorie, plant-based diet.

Many women with breast cancer have, or develop, health conditions that can be improved with a healthy diet, exercise, and achieving a healthy body weight. This includes the improvement in health conditions such as heart disease, diabetes, osteoporosis, and obesity as well as the prevention of other cancers. The good news is that the same lifestyle recommendation for cancer recurrence will benefit women in preventing or improving other health conditions.

Why is a healthy body weight important for women with breast cancer?

A healthy body weight is defined as a body mass index (BMI) in the range of 18.5 to 24.9 km/m2. Achieving and maintaining a healthy body weight is important for women who have been diagnosed with breast cancer for several reasons. A healthy weight may decrease the risk of breast cancer recurrence and improve survival, and it benefits overall health by decreasing the risk of common health conditions such as heart disease, diabetes, and other new cancers.

To calculate your body mass index, see the chart to the right and the table below.

BMI range	Interpretation
Less than 18.5	Underweight
Between 18.5 – 24.9	Ideal
Between 25 – 29.9	Overweight
Greater than 30	Obese

BMI	Height (inches)																		
Weight (lbs.)	58	59	60	61	62	63	64	65	66	67	68	69	70	71	72	73	74	75	76
	4'10"	4'11"	5'0"	5'1"	5'2"	5'3"	5'4"	5'5"	5'6"	5'7"	5'8"	5'9"	5'10"	5'11"	6'0"	6'1"	6'2"	6'3"	6'4"
100	21	20	20	19	18	18	17	17	16	16	15	15	14	14	14	13	13	13	12
105	22	21	21	20	19	19	18	18	17	16	16	16	15	15	14	14	14	13	13
110	23	22	22	21	20	20	19	18	18	17	17	16	16	15	15	15	14	14	13
115	24	23	23	22	21	20	20	19	19	18	18	17	17	16	16	15	15	14	14
120	25	24	23	23	22	21	21	20	19	19	18	18	17	17	16	16	15	15	15
125	26	25	24	24	23	22	22	21	20	20	19	18	18	17	17	17	16	16	15
130	27	26	25	25	24	23	22	22	21	20	20	19	19	18	18	17	17	16	16
135	28	27	26	26	25	24	23	23	22	21	21	20	19	19	18	18	17	17	16
140	29	28	27	27	26	25	24	23	23	22	21	21	20	20	19	19	18	18	17
145	30	29	28	27	27	26	25	24	23	23	22	21	21	20	20	19	19	18	18
150	31	30	29	28	27	27	26	25	24	24	23	22	22	21	20	20	19	19	18
155	32	31	30	29	28	28	27	26	25	24	24	23	22	22	21	20	20	19	19
160	34	32	31	30	29	28	28	27	26	25	24	24	23	22	22	21	21	20	20
165	35	33	32	31	30	29	28	28	27	26	25	24	24	23	22	22	21	21	20
170	36	34	33	32	31	30	29	28	27	27	26	25	24	24	23	22	22	21	21
175	37	35	34	33	32	31	30	29	28	27	27	26	25	24	24	23	23	22	21
180	38	36	35	34	33	32	31	30	29	28	27	27	26	25	24	24	23	23	22
185	39	37	36	35	34	33	32	31	30	29	28	27	27	26	25	24	24	23	23
190	40	38	37	36	35	34	33	32	31	30	29	28	27	27	26	25	24	24	23
195	41	39	38	37	36	35	34	33	32	31	30	29	28	27	27	26	25	24	24
200	42	40	39	38	37	36	34	33	32	31	30	30	29	28	27	26	26	25	24
205	43	41	40	39	38	36	35	34	33	32	31	30	29	29	28	27	26	26	25
210	44	43	41	40	38	37	36	35	34	33	32	31	30	29	29	28	27	26	26
215	45	44	42	41	39	38	37	36	35	34	33	32	31	30	29	28	28	27	26
220	46	45	43	42	40	39	38	37	36	35	34	33	32	31	30	29	28	28	27
225	47	46	44	43	41	40	39	38	36	35	34	33	32	31	31	30	29	28	27
230	48	47	45	44	42	41	40	38	37	36	35	34	33	32	31	30	30	29	28
235	49	48	46	44	43	42	40	39	38	37	36	35	34	33	32	31	30	29	29
240	50	49	47	45	44	43	41	40	39	38	37	36	35	34	33	32	31	30	29
245	51	50	48	46	45	43	42	41	40	38	37	36	35	34	33	32	32	31	30
250	52	51	49	47	46	44	43	42	40	39	38	37	36	35	34	33	32	31	30

What about specific foods such as soy and flaxseed? Are they safe?

At one time, soybeans, flaxseeds, and foods containing them were a concern for women with a history of breast cancer. This is because these foods contain a source of estrogen, known as *plant estrogens* or *phytoestrogens*. New evidence has found that soy foods are safe for breast cancer survivors when eaten in amounts similar to typical Asian diets (two servings per day). From the available evidence it is unclear whether there may be benefits beyond general health for women with breast cancer in terms of lowering the risk of recurrence or improving survival. Also, until more information is available women are advised to avoid soy supplements, such as soy products in concentrated or pill form.

Flaxseeds are a good source of fibre and provide a rich source of fat called *omega 3 fatty acids*. Similar to soy, ground flaxseeds are a source of weak plant estrogens. Flaxseed is safe when used in moderation (1 to 2 tablespoons of ground flaxseed per day) as part of a healthy diet. It is unclear whether there may be benefits beyond general health for women with a history of breast cancer.

Can I drink alcohol if I have had breast cancer?

There is strong evidence that drinking alcohol leads to an increased risk of developing breast cancer. Early evidence also suggests that in women diagnosed with breast cancer, alcohol may also increase the risk of recurrence of breast cancer, but further research is needed. Overall, if you drink alcohol it is prudent to limit consumption to less than one drink per day for women (two drinks per day for men). The risk of breast cancer associated with alcohol applies to all types of alcohol. One serving of an alcoholic beverage is equal one of the following: 145 ml (5 oz) wine, or 350 ml (12 oz) bottle of beer, or 45 ml (1.5 oz) of spirits (whiskey, rye, gin, etc).

Is there a special diet to follow during cancer treatment?

Your body needs a wide variety of nutrients to aid in healing after surgery or while undergoing radiation therapy or chemotherapy. The Healthy Eating Plan for Women at the end of this chapter can be used as a general guide to select foods during treatment and recovery. However, treatment for breast cancer or a recurrence can cause side effects that at times can make it more difficult to eat. Some women experience nausea, vomiting, weight changes, diarrhea (or constipation), a sore mouth or throat, a change in appetite, or a change in the way food tastes. Almost all women will experience fatigue. Modifications to your diet, along with a once-a-day multivitamin and mineral supplement, may be recommended if you are unable to eat a variety of vegetables, fruits, and whole grain foods.

For more information see the Canadian Cancer Society's guidebook *Eating Well When You Have Cancer: A guide to good nutrition* (2008) or visit www.cancer.ca.

If you are having chemotherapy

During chemotherapy, nausea, a sore mouth, taste changes, and mild diarrhea may occur.

Ease nausea with starchy snacks and light drinks

Nausea is best controlled by a combination of medications and certain foods. Dry, starchy foods like crackers and dry cereals, eaten often, help minimize the empty stomach feeling that can make nausea worse.

Fluids like flat ginger ale, weak tea, diluted fruit juice, or ice water are generally better tolerated than milkshakes, coffee, or very sweet juices. Keeping a thermos or large cup close by can help remind you of the importance of drinking lots of fluid during chemotherapy.

If the smell of cooking food makes nausea worse, try to avoid being in the kitchen. If this is not realistic, consider simply prepared or purchased or homemade meals that can be easily reheated.

Soothe mouth sores

If mouth sores occur during chemotherapy, certain foods such as oranges and grapefruit, salty or spicy foods, or rough foods, like toast, should be avoided until the sores heal. Many women find cold foods like fruit, yogurt, ice milk, and blended shakes very soothing.

If foods taste different

Some women notice that certain foods taste different during chemotherapy. For example, meat might taste bitter or metallic. If this happens, high-protein alternatives such as eggs, milk, or tofu will make eating more enjoyable. Food cravings can also occur. Some women crave comfort foods during treatment, whereas others find that fruit and certain vegetables are the most appealing.

Coping with diarrhea and gas

You can minimize diarrhea by limiting your intake of alcohol, strong coffee, strong tea, and cola, and by temporarily eating fewer high-fibre foods such as bran cereals and whole grain breads. Excess gas can be at least partially controlled by eating fewer gas-forming foods such as legumes (beans) and vegetables from the cabbage family, such as cabbage, Brussels sprouts, and broccoli.

If you are having radiation therapy

During radiation, fatigue and a mild sore throat may occur.

If you are feeling tired

The use of convenience or take-out foods, leftovers, or previously prepared and frozen meals can reduce the effort of meal prepara-tion. If possible, arrange to have some meals prepared by family or friends, or use grocery delivery or catering services. As well, simple meals, such as a sandwich or a bowl of cereal with milk and fruit, can also be nutritious.

Sore throat or difficulty swallowing

Women whose radiation treatment involves the throat area sometimes develop temporary soreness or discomfort during swal-lowing. Eating soft, moist foods is helpful, such as hot or cold cereals, soups, pasta, fruit, yogurt, poached eggs, canned fish, or chicken stew. If needed, a smooth consistency can be achieved by putting foods through a blender. Very hot foods such as tea, soup, or spicy foods can make a sore throat worse.

If you are having hormonal therapy

A form of hormonal treatment called *aromotase inhibitors* (see Chapter 28) that lowers the estrogen levels in the body may cause bone loss and over time increase the risk of osteoporosis. Tamoxifen as hormone therapy does not cause this problem. Post-menopausal women and those who experience early menopause due to chemotherapy are at increased risk of bone loss. Bone loss and osteoporosis may be reduced if a woman takes calcium and vitamin D. It is necessary to take both. The calcium is required to build up the bones and the vitamin D is required to lay the calcium into the bones. The recommended amounts of calcium and vitamin D are shown in Table 8.

Table 8 Select women's calcium and vitamin D needs		
Women on hormone therapy at average risk of osteoporosis	**Calcium**	**Vitamin D**
Premenopausal	1200 mg	600 IU
Postmenopausal	1500 mg	800 IU
Women not on hormone therapy but at higher risk of osteoporosis		
Premenopausal	1000 mg	600 IU
Postmenopausal	1200 mg	600 IU

Aside from bone health, vitamin D has some other health benefits. The Canadian Cancer Society recommends a supplement of 1000 IU of vitamin D daily for cancer prevention.

What about gaining weight during treatment?

Regardless of the type of treatment you are receiving, weight gain is common in women with breast cancer. It occurs most often in premenopausal women treated with chemotherapy or hormone therapy. The exact cause of weight gain is unclear, but it could be due to a number of factors including decreased physical activity, eating frequently to control nausea, eating as an antidote to boredom or stress, or because of an increased appetite or food cravings. If you have experienced natural or treatment-related menopause, are taking Megace, or have recently quit smoking, you may also notice that your weight has increased.

How can weight gain be managed?

Weight gain during treatment may put unnecessary stress on the body, reduce energy levels, and delay recovery. Therefore, aim to avoid weight gain and maintain your weight until treatment is completed. You can do this by eating more fruits, vegetables, and whole grains, which are low in calories. Reducing the portion size of food and limiting high-fat foods will also help to achieve or maintain a healthy weight. If frequent eating is necessary to control nausea, low-fat foods such as low-fat crackers, cereal with skim milk, bread and jam, and fruit are good choices.

Being more physically active will also promote weight loss and has a number of other health benefits such as improved mood, sleep, and body image and increased muscle and bone mass. Your doctor or registered dietitian can offer you more individualized advice.

Are extra vitamins and minerals helpful during treatment?

Despite the popularity and common use of vitamin and mineral supplements, it's not yet clear whether their use helps in cancer treatment. Those who support supplement use suggest that they may restore immune function. Although a number of nutrients are required for the immune system (including vitamins A, C, E, B6, beta-carotene, folic acid, zinc, and iron), too much of a good thing is not necessarily better, and can be harmful. For example, too much zinc actually depresses the immune system.

Another popular theory is that the antioxidant vitamins—vitamins C, E, and beta-carotene—are required to help repair cells damaged during cancer treatment. Although foods that are rich in antioxidants (dark green and orange vegetables and a variety of fruits) are recommended as part of a healthy diet, at present there is not enough evidence to indicate that antioxidant supplements are safe and beneficial during cancer treatment. If you are thinking of using vitamin or mineral supplements in high doses during treatment, discuss it with your physician and registered dietitian.

For more information on complementary and alternative therapies see Chapter 44.

Once treatment is complete

Many women notice that they gain weight in the years after a breast cancer diagnosis. Some attribute the weight gain to tamoxifen, but in research studies the amount of weight gain has been similar whether women were taking tamoxifen or placebo. It is unclear what causes weight gain in some women. Overall, we know that weight gain or loss is related to an imbalance between the amount of calories eaten and the energy burned off doing the activities of daily living and additional exercise.

If you have completed your cancer treatment and haven't already made healthful changes to your diet, this is a good time to start. Following a low-fat diet and achieving a healthy body weight may lower the risk of breast cancer recurrence. Eating less fat and more fruit, vegetables, and whole-grain foods can help you regain the sense of control and well being that will enhance your recovery. Besides a possible connection to breast cancer risk, too much fat in the diet has also been linked to the development of heart disease and obesity.

Increasing the emphasis on wholesome and naturally low-fat foods such as whole grains, legumes (beans) and lentils, fruits, and vegetables can reduce the fat in your diet. You can also limit fat by removing visible sources on chicken or meat wherever possible, and by using low-fat cooking methods such as poaching, broiling, and baking. In addition, use less butter, margarine, or mayonnaise on sandwiches and use light salad dressings or extra herbs and spices to flavour food. As you probably know, foods such as crackers, cookies, cakes, potato chips, ice cream, and cheese are generally high in fat. Reading food labels to check the amount of fat is a good idea and will help you choose low-fat alternatives. A registered dietitian can provide further advice.

Ongoing research for unanswered questions

Research in the area of diet and breast cancer is constantly evolving in an attempt to answer many remaining questions such as the effect of diet and exercise on breast cancer recurrence and survival. For example, it is not yet known whether women with a history of breast cancer will benefit from additional vitamin and minerals supplements such as vitamin D. However, healthy eating is always a positive step in general.

Healthy Eating Plan for Women

In one day you should eat:	**Women 19 to 50 years:** Vegetables and fruit = 7 to 8 servings Grain products = 6 to 7 servings Milk and alternatives = 2 servings Meat and alternatives = 2 servings **Women age 51 years or older:** Vegetables and fruit = 7 servings Grain products = 6 servings Milk and alternatives = 3 servings Meat and alternatives = 2 servings
Vegetables and fruit (each is one serving)	· 125 ml (½ cup) vegetables (fresh, frozen, or canned) · 125 ml (½ cup) leafy vegetables (cooked) · 250 ml (1 cup) leafy vegetables (raw) · 1 fruit or 125 ml (½ cup) fruit (fresh, frozen, or canned) · 125 ml (½ cup) 100% juice
Grain products (each is one serving)	· 1 slice (35 g) bread · ½ bagel (45 g) · ½ pita or ½ tortilla (35 g) · 125 ml (½ cup) rice, bulgur, or quinoa (cooked) · 30 g cereal (cold) · 175 ml (¾ cup) cereal (hot) · 125 ml (½ cup) pasta or couscous (cooked)
Meat and alternatives (each is one serving)	· 75 g (2½ oz) or 125 ml (½ cup) fish, shellfish, poultry, or lean meat (cooked) · 175 ml (¾ cup) beans (legumes) (cooked) · 150 g or 175 ml (¾ cup) tofu · 2 eggs · 30 ml (2 Tbsp) peanut or nut butters · 60 ml (¼ cup) nuts and seeds

Healthy Eating Plan for Women

Milk products (each is one serving)	Milk products are an excellent source of calcium. Each serving contains approximately 300 mg of calcium. • 250 ml (1 cup) milk • 125 ml (½ cup) milk (canned, evaporated) • 250 ml (1 cup) fortified soy beverage • 175 g (¾ cup) yogurt • 175 g (¾ cup) Kefir • 50 g (1½ oz) cheese
Other high calcium foods include:	• 8 medium (3½ oz) sardines (canned) • 250 ml (1 cup) calcium-fortified orange juice • 90 g (3 oz) salmon (canned with bones) • 15 ml (1 Tbsp) blackstrap molasses • 60 ml (¼ cup) almonds • 1 medium orange • 2 medium figs (dried) • 125 ml (½ cup) broccoli
Make every serving count:	• Eat at least one dark green and one orange vegetable each day • Choose vegetables and fruit prepared with little or not added fat, sugar, or salt • Have vegetables and fruit more often than juice • Make at least half of your grain products whole grain each day • Choose grain products that are lower in fat, sugar, or salt • Drink skim, 1%, or 2% milk • Select lower-fat milk alternatives • Have meat alternatives such as beans, lentils, and tofu • Eat at least two servings of fish per week • Select lean meat and alternatives prepared with little or no added fat or salt

Adapted from Eating Well with Canada's Food Guide (2007)

More advice on nutrition

The Healthy Eating Plan for Women on the previous two pages, which is adapted from *Eating Well with Canada's Food Guide*, provides a straightforward introduction to healthy eating. You can obtain further advice about nutrition by contacting a registered dietitian at your regional cancer center or community hospital. As well, in some cities there are nutrition hotlines staffed by qualified dietitians. Check with your local dietetic association about resources in your area.

In the United States, the phone number of the Consumer Nutrition Hotline of the American Dietetic Association is 1-800-366-1655. In Canada, a registered dietitian can be contacted at no charge at EatRight Ontario at 1-877-510-510-2 (Ontario residents), or at HealthLinkBC by calling 8-1-1 (British Columbia residents).

The Additional Reading section includes cookbooks devoted to lower fat, higher fibre meals. The recipes are easy to follow and, most importantly, taste great!

CHAPTER THIRTY-SIX

Stress and relaxation

What is stress?

STRESS IS WOVEN INTO THE FABRIC OF LIFE. At healthy levels it challenges us and promotes activity, but when a person feels over-loaded or loses control then the stress is no longer healthy. The uncertainty and fear surrounding a diagnosis of breast cancer can lead to a feeling of overload just when there is a great need to be in control, and it can threaten a person's well being.

How much stress am I feeling?

Stress is a subjective response that is not expressed the same way in each person. When stress becomes too great, the mind may fool you into thinking that you are coping, but the body gives more accurate signals. If you recognize and acknowledge your own stress response, it is easier to deal with it.

To assess your own response to stress, it is helpful to learn to scan your body while asking yourself questions. Start at the top of your head, searching for tightness between your eyebrows. Are your lips pursed? Is your jaw clenched? Are your shoulders hunched up near your ears? Often, we don't notice these things until we are alerted by a pounding headache or lower back pain at the end of the day. Do you feel tightness in the throat, a constriction in the chest or a churning stomach? Are you breathing shallowly, using only the upper part of your chest? Does your heart beat fast? Some people notice that their sleep pattern is disturbed, and others eat more than they need because eating is comforting.

When in distress, the mind doesn't focus and function the way it usually does. You may forget your own telephone number or an important appointment. Your thoughts could become dark and repetitive, and after only an hour's sleep you may lie awake for hours doing what has been so aptly called "awfulizing." Emotionally, you are not as steady as usual, and find yourself in tears over something that you would normally take in stride.

To be told to relax at a time like this seems unreasonable. However, when you are not feeling the effects of an overload of stress, you find yourself filled with a tranquil energy and a sense of control. How do you achieve this elusive feeling, especially after a recent diagnosis of breast cancer?

How can I reduce stress and regain a sense of control?

Reading this book, gaining knowledge about breast cancer, is one practical way to help you find that sense of control. Also, finding someone to listen, though this sounds simple, is of enormous value.

Research has shown that even 20 minutes a day of relaxation can have a beneficial effect on the body. It doesn't matter whether it is transcendental meditation or simply sitting quietly watching the birds at a feeder outside the window. Twenty minutes of steady walking or other exercise works for some people. Tai Chi and yoga also use movement to bring the body and mind into a state of harmony. Meditation teaches us to focus our minds on a particular word (mantra) or object (mandala), or on the rising and falling of the breath to still the chattering mind and restore a sense of equilibrium. Anything that allows the body to be at ease and the mind to become quieter brings back balance and harmony. Think of the ocean. Even when a storm is raging, deep below there is a place where the water is calm. So it is with your own self. You need to find the way down to that place deep within yourself where you are calm and in control, even in the midst of chaos.

Women are used to being responsible for others and putting their own needs last. Giving yourself permission to take some time for yourself can be an important part of the healing process. Be your own good caregiver; and know that it is healthy to say "yes" to your own needs.

The relaxation response

Relaxation is about tranquil energy and gaining a sense of control so that you can respond to situations with good choices. It is interesting that the ancient Chinese symbol for crisis has two components, one meaning "danger," the other meaning "opportunity." Gaining a sense of control gives you an opportunity to make creative choices.

The breath is the pulse of the mind. You can slow your racing thoughts simply by changing your breathing, especially by breathing from the bottom of the diaphragm instead of the shallow, tight breathing from high in the chest that usually accompanies stress. For example: take a comfortable, deep breath, hold it to the count of four and then let it out with a sigh. Repeat this four times. Feel how your shoulders release and your facial muscles soften. When you find yourself experiencing tension, remind yourself to take a sighing breath.

"Autogenics" is another way to occupy the thinking mind by getting it busy with repeated words such as "My right arm is heavy, my right arm is warm." With this repetition, the mind starts to convince the body that its different parts are at ease. This feeling of bodily comfort induces a sense of calm control.

Another way to achieve the relaxation response is to imagine yourself in a beautiful place, perhaps in nature or a delightful room, or to relive the memory of a time of achievement and strength. This is the opposite of "awfulizing," as you use your body-mind connection to create sensations of peace and connectedness. Audio recordings can also be very helpful by coaching you through these experiences (see Additional Reading).

Quick fixes

Sometimes finding even 20 minutes a day for relaxation seems like a tall order. In this case, experiment with some quick fixes to help familiarize you with the healing benefits of relaxation.

Whenever you are particularly stressed you quite naturally do one of these quick fixes already: you sigh. You can cultivate sighing as a way towards relaxation. After three or four comfortable sighing breaths you will find that the muscles of the face are more at ease, the chest feels more open and the shoulders are softer. Because one needs regular reminders to sigh, try putting little coloured dots in all sorts of places such as on your steering wheel, on the telephone, or on your purse. These dots can serve as triggers, reminders to take a breath, hold it to the count of four, and then sigh the breath out. Do this throughout the day.

Another quick fix is to practice a quick progressive muscle relaxation every time you sit down. Let tension flow from the top of your head out through the soles of your feet. Or take a 30-second vacation and recall a beautiful place or happy, carefree time.

Certain fragrances are known to soothe and elevate one's mood. Try a few drops of neroli oil, lavender, geranium, or another fragrance that pleases you as you relax in a warm bath. Many health food stores and pharmacies carry aromatherapy products.

Increasingly, you will recognize the importance of your own role in the healing process in partnership with your physicians and their treatments and medications. Learning your role can add a rich dimension to the power of this partnership.

What if cancer recurs?

CHAPTER THIRTY-SEVEN

Follow-up: Support, side effects, and concerns about recurrence

OFTEN, IT IS ONLY AT THE END OF TREATMENT that women start to worry about the possibility of a relapse. "What if the breast cancer recurs? When will it recur? What can I do to prevent it from coming back? What is my prognosis if it does relapse? Will I die? How long have I got?" Understandably, these disturbing questions can plague the mind.

What are the goals of follow-up?

There are several purposes of regular follow-up after treatment for breast cancer including providing support, to assess, to explain and manage any side effects from treatment, and to offer early detection of potentially curable recurrent or new disease. Follow-up visits also give you an opportunity to ask questions and discuss any new information you are wondering about. Unfortunately, although there are many useful treatments should breast cancer recur, there is yet no curative treatment if breast cancer is found in organs beyond the breast and lymph node regions. Therefore, the doctors focus on looking for potentially curable new disease in the breast or lymph nodes with physical examinations and regular mammograms. If a woman has no symptoms, there is no value in doing tests such as chest X-rays, bone scans, or blood tests to determine if breast cancer has spread to other organs.

What are the chances of a recurrence?

Recurrences happen because cancer cells were not removed or were resistant to the initial treatment. Recurrence may be local if it occurs in the skin of the chest wall, breast, or regional if it occurs in the lymph nodes. Recurrences are called *systemic* when they occur in other parts of the body such as the bones, liver, lungs, or brain. *Metastasize* refers to the movement of cancer cells. A new growth of the breast cancer in organs beyond the breast is called a *metastasis*.

The risk of recurrence is related to several factors, including whether the cancer is in situ or invasive, the type of cancer (is it hormone sensitive or HER2 positive?), the size of the tumour, and the presence and number of cancer-involved lymph nodes. Patients with only in situ disease have a very low risk of the cancer recurring elsewhere in the body, but there is a possibility of local recurrence in the treated breast or of a cancer developing in the other breast.

For women with invasive cancers, the risk of relapse is related to the type of the primary cancer (see Chapter 12) and the extent or stage of disease at the time of diagnosis (see Chapter 16). Patients with stage I disease (a small tumour, with no cancer found in the axillary lymph nodes), are unlikely to have a recurrence and have an 85 to 95% of being alive and free of disease 10 years or more after treatment, especially if the cancer was low grade. In more advanced stages, the risk of relapse is greater. Approximately 40% of stage II patients and 60% of those with a stage III cancer will develop a recurrence either locally or elsewhere in the body within 10 years of treatment.

New therapies for breast cancer are being studied all over the world and the information from these studies is shared internationally in an attempt to improve cure rates. It is hoped that over the next few years fewer women will suffer a relapse.

When should I worry about a new problem?

Most recurrences beyond the breast cause symptoms; they are rarely silent. The symptoms depend on which organ is affected. For example, breast cancer that has travelled to the bones will often cause bone pain, while recurrences in the lungs may cause cough or shortness of breath. It is often difficult for a patient who has recently been diagnosed to know which symptoms might indicate recurrent disease and which symptoms are simply normal aches and pains. It takes time for a woman to start trusting her body again after a diagnosis of breast cancer. Worry about relapse makes it hard to be at ease.

In general, symptoms of recurrence are more persistent than normal aches and pains and become progressively worse. For example, a backache brought on by moving furniture usually feels bad for a day or two and then gradually gets better. Metastatic breast cancer to a bone in the back may come on gradually, may come and go with activity and may respond to painkillers, but it will not go away completely and stay away. Instead, it will become more persistent. If you are worried about a new symptom, especially if it is persistent or getting worse, you should see your doctor. She or he will do an examination and order any necessary tests. If everything is normal and the symptoms continue to bother you, they could be caused by something other than the breast cancer. Naturally, not all new symptoms mean a recurrence of breast cancer, but your doctor should do an evaluation and arrive at a diagnosis.

How and by whom should I be followed?

All women, after a diagnosis of breast cancer, should have follow-up visits to provide information and support and to check for a local recurrence or new cancer in the opposite breast. However, medical opinion differs on the best follow-up schedule, and women's needs also vary. Some women are comfortable with frequent follow-up and the reassurance that there is no detectable recurrence. Other women find that follow-up visits cause unnecessary anxiety. The woman and her doctor should agree on a schedule of follow-up that provides reassurance and support and detects most recurrences promptly, but allows the woman to return to normal living.

It is not essential that you be followed at a cancer centre. Most women receive excellent support and surveillance from their family physicians. It is important that you feel confident in the doctor's ability to listen to you and examine you, particularly the treated breast if you have had breast-conserving surgery. If you are seeing several different physicians, space out the visits to avoid duplication.

There is very little advantage to the early detection of recurrence beyond the breast or lymph nodes because currently available treatments for metastatic disease are not curative. Therefore performing X-rays, scans, or blood tests to look for metastatic disease is not recommended unless there is some new, worrisome symptom that needs to be checked. As well, unnecessary X-rays expose you to unnecessary radiation. However, local treatment (surgery, radiation, or both) may be curative for a local recurrence or a new cancer developing in the opposite breast. Surveillance mammograms are usually the best way to detect new disease in the breast tissue. Therefore, regular mammograms are the only routine test recommended for a woman who otherwise feels well in the years following breast cancer treatment. In women with a very high risk of developing a new breast cancer after the first one, such as those with a hereditary risk, breast MRIs may also be done.

How often should I have follow-up visits and what should happen at the visit?

We recommend a first follow-up visit about 6 to 8 weeks after the initial surgery, chemotherapy, and radiation therapy are complete. Then, you should have visits approximately every 3 to 6 months for the first 3 years and then every 6 to 12 months until year 5. After 5 years, an annual checkup is recommended. At each visit, the physician should ask about your level of appetite, energy, menopausal symptoms, pain, arm swelling, and your emotional health as well as check whether you are taking and tolerating any medications (such as hormone therapy) that may have been prescribed. You should expect to be examined, at least in the region of the breasts, arms, neck, chest, and abdomen. This visit should also be an opportunity for you to ask questions. Be sure to tell your doctor about any new symptoms or changes in how your body is functioning including aches and pains in bones, any persistent cough or shortness of breath, nausea, weight loss, or new lumps or bumps. Any of these symptoms could possibly be indications of recurrent disease. You should also discuss your psychological and lifestyle issues, side effects from any medications, and report any menopausal or hormonal concerns including vaginal discharge, dryness, or bleeding.

Blood tests are often normal despite evidence of a local or even distant recurrence and are *not* recommended as part of regular checkups. Routine bone or liver scans, chest X-rays, or tests other than annual mammograms are *not* recommended in women without symptoms. X-rays, scans, and blood tests might be done if a woman has noticed a new symptom or change in her body.

The important thing is whether you have symptoms. If you have none, the only regular tests you need are mammograms and physical examinations. However, any new or persistent symptom should be investigated.

Mammograms

If you had breast conserving surgery, it is strongly recommended that you have a baseline mammogram approximately 6 months after the completion of the surgery, chemotherapy, or radiation therapy, whichever is the last treatment, or within a year of your previous mammogram. If you had a mastectomy then there is no value in doing a mammogram of the mastectomy side but having an annual mammogram of the other breast is recommended.

It is highly unlikely that cancer recurrence will be detected on a baseline mammogram done 6 months after surgery and radiation therapy. By then however, most of the breast changes due to treatment should have settled and a mammogram at that time can serve as a new normal to be used for comparison with future mammograms. Subsequently, mammograms should be done once each year. Not all mammogram abnormalities after treatment are cancer. After surgery and radiation therapy there may be changes in the breast such as scarring or swelling, which can be monitored with regular mammograms. Mammograms of the unaffected breast should be performed once a year because over 10 years of follow-up, between 3 and 5% of women develop a new cancer in the other breast.

Ultrasound and MRI of the breast

Ultrasounds and MRIs may be helpful if there is something that is not clearly seen on the mammogram, but are not recommended as part of the routine follow-up after breast cancer treatment. MRIs may also be recommended if you have a familial cancer risk or very dense breast tissue.

Your responsibilities

You are responsible for some aspects of the follow-up. You may want to learn how to do breast self-examination. This includes examining the uninvolved breast and the radiated breast or the chest wall if a mastectomy has been done. Any new findings or changes should be reported to your doctor. It's important to know that not all changes are due to cancer recurrence. Many women develop thickened areas or redness in a radiated breast, or thickened areas along the scar. Often, it is difficult to know if the thickening is cancerous or not, and a mammogram or biopsy may be necessary. You should show your doctor the area of concern and he or she will do a physical examination and order additional tests if necessary. You should remember to tell any new physicians of your history of breast cancer.

If you notice a new, persisting symptom, make an appointment to see your doctor—don't wait for the next routine appointment if it is more than a few weeks away. If you are not satisfied that the symptom has been explained, insist on a return visit to your oncologist. Specific information about the treatment of local recurrence or recurrence elsewhere in the body are described in Chapters 38 and 39.

CHAPTER THIRTY-EIGHT

Treatment of a local or regional recurrence

A LOCAL OR REGIONAL RECURRENCE refers to a relapse of breast cancer in the breast, the armpit, the skin or muscles of the chest wall, or the surrounding lymph nodes. When the cancer recurs in these areas it is because cancer cells present in the skin, muscles, or lymphatic system were not removed at the time of mastectomy or partial mastectomy and were not killed by any subsequent radiation, chemotherapy, or hormonal treatments (if they were used).

What are the signs of local or regional recurrences?

Possible signs of local or regional relapse include new lumps, thickening or rashes in the breast, chest wall, armpit, or above the collarbone. Recurrence in the lymph nodes in the armpit or behind the collarbone may cause shoulder pain or arm swelling. A new pain that shoots down the arm, or numbness and weakness in the hand or arm may be due to cancer pinching the nerves that extend down into the hand and arm from the neck. See your physician if you have any of these symptoms.

How are local recurrences treated?

Local relapses often require local treatments such as surgery or radiation therapy, especially if there is no evidence of recurrence elsewhere in the body. However, if there is evidence that cancer has also recurred elsewhere in the body, the recurrence may be better treated with systemic treatment such as chemotherapy or hormones. The local relapse should be biopsied to determine whether it is a regrowth of the original cancer or a new cancer, and to confirm the ER and HER2 status, which may influence treatment options.

It is not known whether chemotherapy added to surgery and/or radiation will cure more women with local relapse than surgery and/or radiation alone. Although studies of women in this circumstance have not shown a definite benefit of adding chemotherapy, if the woman is young and has not had previous chemotherapy, it is reasonable to consider the use of chemotherapy after the local recurrence has been removed. If the recurrence is found to be hormone sensitive, and the woman is not on hormone therapy, it may be recommended. If the recurrence is HER2 positive, chemotherapy and an anti-HER2 treatment such as Herceptin may be recommended.

Cancer recurrence in the breast after partial mastectomy and radiation

Cancer may recur in the breast after conservative surgery and radiation in approximately 2 to 10% of women within 10 years of treatment. Usually, recurrence in the breast can be treated for cure, but this often requires a mastectomy. It is usually not possible to repeat a course of radiation if it was used after the initial surgery. To detect small, curable recurrences, we recommend that a physical examination and mammogram be done at least every year, starting about 6 months after completion of the initial surgery, chemotherapy, and radiation therapy.

The primary treatment for a small local recurrence is to remove it with surgery if possible. If the local recurrence is too extensive, chemotherapy and hormones are used prior to surgery. Chemotherapy may also be recommended if the woman is young and did not receive chemotherapy at the time of initial diagnosis or if the recurrence is HER2 positive.

If a local recurrence occurs after partial mastectomy when radiation was not used at the time of initial diagnosis, the cancer re-growth should be removed and radiation therapy should then be given in a further attempt to save the breast.

Treatment of a local or regional recurrence after mastectomy

Recurrence of breast cancer on the chest wall or in lymph nodes in the armpit (axilla), above the collarbone (supraclavicular fossa) or behind the breast bone (internal mammary nodes) may occur following mastectomy. If you have not previously received radiation therapy, the usual treatment is to remove the recurrence surgically (if it is small and localized) and then give radiation therapy (see Chapter 25). If the recurrence is very extensive, with growth into adjacent bones, muscles, or nerves, or cancer recurs within the chest wall and lymph glands after previous radiation therapy, or if recurrence is found at the same time in other organs such as in the lungs or liver, treatment needs to be individualized. In these situations it is usual to use hormones or chemotherapy as the first approach depending on the woman's symptoms, the tumour's ER status, and the type of previous treatment she received.

CHAPTER THIRTY-NINE

Treatment of recurrence elsewhere in the body (metastasis)

Why does the cancer recur elsewhere?

CANCER COMES BACK ELSEWHERE in the body (a *systemic recurrence*) because breast cancer cells escaped into the blood stream prior to the first treatment. Although adjuvant chemotherapy and hormone therapy may have been given to try to destroy these cells, it is not always effective. Cells that are resistant to treatment are not killed and may divide and grow into detectable cancer metastases.

What can I expect if I have a recurrence elsewhere?

The behaviour of the returning cancer depends on a number of factors, including:
- The amount of time passed since the original cancer was diagnosed: a longer time means the recurrence will tend to grow more slowly
- The type of initial cancer: the less aggressive, the better
- The tumour's estrogen receptor status: estrogen receptor-positive tumours tend to grow more slowly
- The number of tumour sites: the fewer, the better
- The sites of the metastases: for example, bone metastases are often slower growing than liver metastases
- The physical state of the woman

The most important factor, however, is how the cancer responds to therapy. If the cancer responds to one type of treatment, then it is more likely that other treatments will also be effective. If the cancer does not shrink in response to any of the usual treatments, the outlook is not as good.

What are the signs of systemic recurrence?

The most common sites for breast cancer to spread are the bones, lungs, liver, and brain. Other parts of the body may also be affected including the lymph nodes, skin, eyes, spinal cord, and ovaries. When breast cancer spreads, the cells still look and behave like the original breast cancer. Therefore, if a breast cancer spreads to the lung, it is still breast cancer (not lung cancer). This is important because the types of treatment and the chance of success are different for a spreading breast cancer than, for instance, a lung cancer.

The symptoms of breast cancer metastases depend on the part of the body affected. Cancer in the bones usually causes progressively increasing pain or a spontaneous fracture (a broken bone). In the lungs, it may cause cough or shortness of breath. In the liver it causes loss of appetite, pain in the right upper abdomen, and sometimes jaundice. If cancer spreads to the brain it may cause headache, numbness or weakness of an arm or leg, loss of balance, confusion, or seizures.

This list of potential problems may be frightening, and a woman may find herself constantly checking for new problems. This is quite normal. The important things to report are persistent changes. Symptoms that come and go within 24 hours are not a sign of cancer.

What are the goals of treatment of recurrence?

The goals of treatment of metastatic breast cancer are to relieve symptoms, maintain quality of life, and prolong survival. The word *cure* comes up with hopes for a successful treatment of the systemic recurrence. However, disappointment often follows when the physician cannot guarantee or even predict promising results. Many people live with longstanding (chronic) diseases that cannot be cured, such as heart disease, emphysema, diabetes, and arthritis. Treatment for those conditions is not curative but is given to help avoid severe complications and symptoms. Metastatic breast cancer can be similar to one of these chronic diseases, with a series of treatments given to decrease the symptoms and avoid complications. After a systemic recurrence, breast cancer is usually not curable. However, the length of life can be years and it is impossible to accurately predict how long a particular individual may survive. The average survival after the cancer travels to an organ is about 2 years, but many women live much longer.

The treatments

If the recurrent cancer can be biopsied, this should be done to assess the characteristics of the cancer as that may determine the treatment. For example, if the cancer is sensitive to estrogens, hormone therapy may be the first treatment. Patients with metastatic breast cancer usually receive a sequence of treatments, including hormones, radiotherapy, chemotherapy, nutritional support, pain management, psychological support, and sometimes surgery.

Systemic (whole body) therapy with hormones or chemotherapy may be recommended. The type of systemic therapy used depends on a number of factors:

- The type of the original tumour: whether it was estrogen or progesterone receptor-positive and/or HER2 overexpressing and the type of cancer in the recurrence (if it has been biopsied).
- The length of time since the original diagnosis: even if the initial tumour was estrogen receptor-negative a recurrence occurring many years later may suggest a hormone-responsive cancer.
- The organs involved: bone metastases may respond better to hormones.
- The severity of the symptoms: if the recurrence is widespread and causing a lot of symptoms then the patient needs a more rapid response and chemotherapy may be recommended. Response to hormone therapy may take a few months so would not be a good choice if the cancer was rapidly growing.
- The age of the patient: chemotherapy may be too harsh for an elderly woman with other health problems.
- The response to previous therapies: if one hormone therapy had a benefit others may too.

- If the cancer was HER2 positive Herceptin may be given along with chemotherapy or possibly hormone therapy.

When is hormone therapy used?

For most systemic recurrences the first therapy used is hormones, especially if the original breast cancer was estrogen-receptor positive. Even if the original cancer was estrogen receptor-negative, if a few years have passed since that diagnosis, the cancer may respond. In this situation a biopsy of the recurrent tumour may help define the best treatment. The therapies with the fewest side effects are used first, followed by ones that are less well tolerated. Tumours that respond and shrink may stay stable for a long time, especially with hormone therapy, but at some point may again progress. If there has been a good response to the initial therapy and the cancer regrows, the initial hormone therapy will be stopped and a new hormone will be tried.

For postmenopausal women, hormonal therapy is usually the first treatment often with an aromatase inhibitor followed by tamoxifen, faslodex, or other hormones (see Chapter 28). Premenopausal women may be treated with tamoxifen, removal of her ovaries, or with hormone agents that block the ovarian function. If a premenopausal woman becomes menopausal, aromatase inhibitors may be used.

When is chemotherapy used?

Chemotherapy is used as the first treatment for a systemic recurrence when the tumour is not likely to respond to hormones. This may include a fast-growing tumour, one that occurs soon after the initial diagnosis, or if the original cancer was estrogen receptor-negative. Chemotherapy is also used to treat cancers that have not responded to a trial of hormone therapy or those that initially responded to hormones but are no longer doing so. Chemotherapy with Herceptin is commonly used in HER2 overexpressing tumours.

For how long is chemotherapy continued?

In recurrent disease, chemotherapy is usually given for two or three cycles and the response is then assessed. If the cancer is responding then treatment may be continued for as long as there is evidence of response and the toxicity is tolerable. If there is not a good response to the first few cycles of chemotherapy, a second type may be tried. If the cancer does not respond to two different types of chemotherapy, it is clearly a very resistant cancer. In this situation the oncologist may decide to avoid further chemotherapy if it is causing side effects and appears to be of no benefit.

Often, chemotherapy can effectively decrease the symptoms of metastatic cancer, such as the shortness of breath that may occur if the cancer is in the lungs. It can also reduce symptoms from bone involvement, enlarged lymph nodes, tumours of the skin or liver, or tumours in the abdomen. Unfortunately it can rarely overcome the fatigue that is a common complaint of women with recurrent cancer.

Studies have evaluated high-dose chemotherapy and bone marrow transplants as treatments for women with systemic recurrences. The studies suggest that these strategies are not an improvement over standard-dose chemotherapy, and should not be used except in a research study.

When is radiation used to treat systemic recurrences?

Radiation may be given for recurrent tumours that cause symptoms in a specific area of the body. This includes recurrence in the lymph nodes in the chest that cause shortness of breath, tumours near the esophagus that interfere with swallowing, or tumours in the bones, brain, and other structures.

The decision to treat with radiation is based on several factors: the site of the recurrence, the symptoms that may be relieved by the treatment, the symptoms that may be caused by the treatment, and how much radiation, if any, the area has received in the past. Organs in the body tolerate radiation differently. Some areas can only be treated once or can only tolerate low doses of radiation, while other areas, such as the bones, can be re-treated or given high doses.

Radiation may be given together with hormones, chemotherapy and/or Herceptin, or by itself. Radiation is often very successful to decrease pain, particularly bone pain. The relief from pain occurs because radiation kills cancer cells, causing tumours to shrink, relieving pressure in the bones. The pain relief may be immediate (a day or two) or gradual (over a month or so). Bones can tolerate high doses of radiation, so if radiation relieved pain once but the pain returns in the same area, the radiation may be repeated with benefit.

The mainstay of treatment for a cancer that recurs in the brain is radiation to the whole brain. The side effects of this therapy include fatigue, mild nausea, and headaches, which can usually be relieved or prevented with low doses of steroids. Hair loss always occurs when the whole brain is treated with radiation, but it begins to grow back after 3 or 4 months. If the patient has a solitary brain metastasis, there may be benefit in having it removed prior to radiation therapy.

Occasionally, if a patient has very widespread cancer in the bones and other attempts to gain control have failed, it may be possible to use an agent called strontium. This is a radioactive material, given intravenously, that settles in bones and can deliver a whole body dose of radiation. The safety and chance of benefit depends on the health of the bone marrow and the degree of bone activity seen on a bone scan.

Can surgery be used to treat systemic recurrences?

If there are bone metastases, surgery to insert pins or plates may be used to stabilize the bone to avoid fractures, to mend bones that have already broken, and to decrease pain. Occasionally, surgery may be used to remove a lump or recurrence on the skin even when there is evidence of other metastases.

If the woman is in reasonable overall shape and has only one site of metastatic disease, surgery can be used to remove it from the lungs, liver, or brain, especially in cases of slow-growing tumours. With breast cancer, however, it is rare to have just a single metastasis, so very few patients are considered for this treatment. Since the cancer cells travel in the blood stream, the surgical removal of a single visible lump will not likely cure the cancer because other, smaller clusters of cells that are still too small to be seen are quite likely to be present elsewhere in the body.

Studies have shown that if there is a solitary metastasis in the brain, doing surgery to remove it if it is easily accessible and then delivering radiation improves symptom relief and survival compared to radiation alone. The decision to do brain surgery for a woman with metastatic breast cancer needs to be considered carefully. This will involve consultation with a neurosurgeon and radiation oncologist who will consider the tumour's location in the brain and the status of the cancer in the rest of the body.

Another local treatment is chemoablation or radiofrequency

ablation of liver metastases and occasionally other sites such as in the lungs. This involves a radiologist inserting a catheter into the liver or affected organ and injecting medication directly into the tumour or delivering high-energy radio waves that heat the tumour to the point of "cooking." Although this technique may shrink the liver tumour, it has some side effects, and does not treat any breast cancer cells outside the liver.

Treatment of fluid accumulation

Recurrent breast cancer can cause excessive fluid to accumulate around the lungs (pleural effusion) due to blockage of normal lymphatic drainage. This can cause shortness of breath or a sharp chest pain that worsens when taking a deep breath. It is usually treated with a chest tube to drain the fluid. Once the fluid is gone, a drug (often doxycycline or bleomycin) or talcum powder is put into the pleural space to close it and prevent the fluid from reaccumulating. This can be done in the operating room or at the bedside. Sometimes a tube (a Pleurex tube) will be put in and left in for the woman or a home care nurse to drain at home on a regular basis.

Fluid may also accumulate in the abdomen and cause an uncomfortable swelling of the belly. If the fluid causes discomfort, temporary relief can be obtained if a catheter is inserted into the abdomen to drain the fluid. However, the fluid usually accumulates again very quickly unless some other treatment of the cancer is given, such as chemotherapy or hormone treatment.

Treatment of bone metastases

Breast cancer commonly involves the bone when it relapses. Drugs known as bisphosphanates have been shown to decrease pain, the need for radiation, and progression of the bone metastases. These may be given orally (clodronate) or intravenously (pamidronate, zolendronic acid) and are often given on a regular basis either as soon as bone recurrence is diagnosed or after there are symptoms. A new drug, denosumab, is a subcutaneous drug (injected under the skin) that has been shown to be effective in decreasing bone-related events. Radiation may decrease pain and be used for specific bone sites. Surgery may be used to stabilize a bone area or treat a fracture.

What can you do for yourself?

Nutrition

Good nutrition is important to maintain a sense of well being, but studies have not shown that diet alone can treat metastatic cancer. For many women with a recurrence, eating becomes difficult because they are fatigued or nauseated. In this situation, a registered dietitian may have useful ideas about how to maintain an adequate diet. Chapter 35 discusses some of these issues.

Pain management

Pain may be present during recurrent breast cancer. Radiation and systemic therapy may provide relief, but using regular and adequate pain medications to avoid letting the pain build up is also important. You will need to find a drug—or cocktail of drugs—that you tolerate well. With a physician's guidance you can increase the dose until the pain is relieved.

Many patients are uneasy about taking medications for pain, especially narcotics, because they are worried that the pills may be addictive or they feel that taking medication for pain is a sign of "giving in." These thoughts are common. Most people will not become addicted to medications that are given to treat pain, and since being pain-free is essential for a good quality of life, it is not a weakness or a sign of giving in to treat the pain. It is simply allowing you to continue as many activities as possible for as long as possible. Unfortunately, all painkillers have side effects. Narcotic medications (codeine, morphine, and others) commonly cause constipation. This can be avoided by taking stool softeners and adequate dietary fibre and fluids as soon as the narcotic medication is started. Bone pain is sometimes decreased by using bisphosphanates (clodronate, pamidronate, etc.).

Mental well being

Psychological well being is also an important part of the treatment of recurrent disease. The support of friends and family is crucial, and individual counselling or discussion with a group of women with recurrent cancer may provide a further means of support. Relaxation groups, massage therapy, or other types of therapy may also help you cope with this new and frightening situation (see Chapter 36).

Clinical trials

Many women with recurrent or advanced cancer are eligible and are approached to participate in research studies (see Chapter 45). This is a common setting to test new drugs or treatments. Carefully consider the options. Many times, a standard therapy is given with the addition of a new drug that is being tested. The risks of participating are that there may be more side effects and the new drug may not be beneficial. The benefits of participating may be getting a new, more effective treatment that is only available as part of the research study and being part of the development of new treatments for women with breast cancer.

Palliative and hospice care

Palliative care concentrates on relieving the symptoms caused by the cancer rather than treating the cancer itself. Many centres have specialized palliative care teams that provide in-hospital and home care support. These teams work cooperatively with the patient and her family to maintain an optimal quality of life. The goals of palliative and hospice care are for the woman to remain comfortable and active with a minimum of symptoms for as long as possible and to enable the woman's independence, dignity, and choices during the difficult final phase of her life. Particular attention is paid to pain relief, nutrition, bowel care, psychological support, and family needs. In many cases good hospice care and adequate resources can allow a woman to stay in her home setting for as long as possible.

Sadly, the reality is that most women with metastatic breast cancer eventually die of their cancer. Frank discussions between the woman and her family to address her desires regarding her death are important. Decisions such as where she may want to die, funeral arrangements, and wills should be made. It is usually better for both the woman and her family to deal with these issues well ahead of the time of need. It is also helpful to discuss how the woman's partner or family are feeling or what they will do after she is gone. Knowing that these matters have been addressed can sometimes offer a certain peace of mind to all of those involved.

Special topics

CHAPTER FORTY

Breast cancer and pregnancy

PREGNANCY ASSOCIATED BREAST CANCER is defined as a breast cancer that is diagnosed during a pregnancy or within 1 year of delivery. Breast cancer can occur during and right after a pregnancy and may be missed as the breasts are engorged and can be difficult to examine.

If breast cancer is diagnosed during pregnancy

If a breast lump or change appears to only one breast during pregnancy, the procedure for diagnosing breast cancer is generally the same as for those who are not pregnant, but extra care is taken to protect the fetus from radiation exposure. Ultrasounds and core biopsies can be done. Mammography can be done with proper shielding of the fetus if necessary. Whole body bone scans should be avoided.

Deciding on a treatment plan

A number of special factors must be considered when treating breast cancer during pregnancy, including the type of the breast cancer, the stage of the cancer, the type of treatment required, and the gestational age of the fetus. The goal of treatment is to have a good result for both the mother and the baby.

In general, surgical therapy (mastectomy, lumpectomy, and axillary dissection) is safe and can proceed. In some circumstances mastectomy is appropriate, with adjuvant treatment delayed until after the birth. Studies have shown that some chemotherapy drugs can be safely given in pregnancy without harming the fetus. The drugs are safer, however, in the later stages (second and third trimester.) Occasionally, if the cancer is progressing very rapidly, a small risk of harm to the fetus may be accepted and chemotherapy or radiotherapy may be started, even while the fetus is still growing.

An obstetric evaluation should be done to determine the exact age of the fetus and to help decide on the best time for delivery. If the fetus is 32 weeks or older, delivery should be done before any chemotherapy or radiation therapy starts. A delay in treatment of about 4 weeks is unlikely to affect the mother's chances of cure, and will allow the baby to mature and have a better chance of being born healthy.

If it is early in the pregnancy, termination may be discussed. Termination does not have an effect on the cancer but may allow earlier treatment with chemotherapy and radiation and in some cases may lessen anxiety for the woman by allowing her to focus on the cancer without fears for her baby.

Some facts about breast cancer and pregnancy

Breast cancer during pregnancy is generally no more aggressive than breast cancer in women of the same age who are not pregnant. The survival of women with breast cancer discovered during pregnancy is similar to survival of other women diagnosed at the same age. However, breast cancer in very young women (younger than 35 years) tends to be more difficult to cure and it can be harder to diagnose during pregnancy, so the breast cancer may be more advanced and may therefore have a higher chance of recurrence. Breast cancer does not spread to the fetus. Abortion of the fetus does not improve the outcome or have an effect on the growth of the mother's cancer.

Is fertility affected by breast cancer treatment?

Premenopausal women who receive chemotherapy may have their menstrual periods stop permanently and they may become infertile. This is more likely to occur as a woman gets older and nears the time of her normal menopause. It is also dependent on the type of chemotherapy that is given. Approximately 30% of women younger than 40 years will have permanent menopause after 6 months of chemotherapy; for women over age 45, permanent menopause is nearly certain after the same treatment. Sometimes menstruation returns 6 months to a year or more after chemotherapy is completed. Since many women remain fertile while receiving chemotherapy, it is important to use effective methods of contraception (but not birth control pills) if you are sexually active. Radiation, unless it is directed at the pelvis, will not affect fertility. Tamoxifen (hormone therapy) may cause menstrual irregularities but does not make women infertile. It is crucial that women use effective contraception while taking tamoxifen because tamoxifen can harm the fetus.

Even if your menstrual periods are not affected, it is recommended that you do not get pregnant until at least 6 months after completing treatment, and that you discuss this with your oncologist. Most of the residual effects of chemotherapy and radiation should have resolved by 6 months.

Pregnancy after breast cancer

Women who get pregnant after having breast cancer have the same long-term cancer outcome as women of the same age who have had breast cancer and do not become pregnant. There is no convincing evidence that getting pregnant makes the cancer regrow or spread any more frequently or faster than if the woman does not get pregnant. Babies born to women who have had treatment for breast cancer in the past do not seem to have any increased chance of fetal malformations or miscarriages.

Following radiation therapy of the breast, the normal breast tissue is permanently altered. The normal engorgement in preparation for lactation does not occur, and during lactation very little, if any, milk is produced from a radiation-treated breast. This means that the breasts may become quite lopsided during pregnancy as the normal breast enlarges and the radiated breast does not. However, breastfeeding from the unaffected breast is still possible and is encouraged.

Making the decision about whether to become pregnant after breast cancer

Apart from the biological considerations, a woman and her partner need to consider various social, psychological, and economic implications of bearing a child. This is doubly hard when the mother-to-be is uncertain of her future. Often, delaying pregnancy for at least 6 months or more after breast cancer treatment is a good idea. This time gives the woman's body and mind a chance to heal. Some doctors recommend a delay of 2 to 5 years to have greater confidence that the cancer won't recur.

CHAPTER FORTY-ONE

Breast cancer in young women

IN RECENT YEARS there has been increased awareness of the specific issues that affect young women who are diagnosed with breast cancer. Breast cancer can occur at any age but is much less common in young women. About 20% of breast cancers occur in women younger than age 50, and only 5% occur in women younger than age 40. The age of 35 is often used as a cutoff for the definition of "young" women as this group tends to have worse prognosis cancers. Some studies have used age 40 years, 50 years, or menopause to define "young" age.

All young women should have a detailed family history taken as the rates of inherited mutations may be higher in young women presenting with breast cancer. It is important that both the mother and father's family history be questioned for breast or ovarian cancer, as inherited tendencies to cancer can be passed down from either side of the family. Genetic testing may be helpful in determining other risks and treatments (see Chapter 42).

Are cancers in young women different?

All types of breast cancer can occur at any age, but high-grade and aggressive cancers are more commonly seen in young women. Young women often have "triple negative" cancers that do not have estrogen or progesterone receptors or HER2 over-expression (see

Chapter 12). Triple negative cancers tend to grow rapidly and are generally treated with chemotherapy. A high-grade tumour in an older woman is also considered aggressive and treated in a similar fashion with chemotherapy. Young women may also present with HER2 over-expressing tumours, and if so are usually treated with chemotherapy and trastuzamab (Herceptin). Young women may present with a type of tumour called a *phylloides tumour*, which is generally treated with surgery alone.

Is the survival of young women different?

Some studies have suggested that the survival of women younger than age 35 is not as good as older women and that younger women have a higher risk of developing distant recurrence. However these statistics may be out of date. Many cancers in young women are high-grade, aggressive cancers (see Chapter 12), and with newer treatments, including trastuzumab for HER2 over-expressing tumours, the survival of these cancers has improved. As well, in the past hormonal therapy was often not given to young women and this may have resulted in poorer outcomes.

What about the local recurrence rate of young women?

There have been studies that show that the local recurrence rate of cancers is higher in young women. This may be related to aggressive tumours or a tendency for younger women to develop multiple tumours in the breast. Studies have shown that giving extra radiation therapy as a boost over the part of the breast where the cancer first started will decrease the risk of local recurrence. A boost dose of radiation therapy is therefore standard among younger women who have been treated with a breast-saving operation (see Chapter 25).

Some oncologists are concerned about the long-term risks of radiation or a higher risk of local recurrence in women younger than age 40 years and may recommend a mastectomy rather than a partial mastectomy followed by radiation therapy. The available studies show that although younger women do have a higher risk of local recurrence than older women, this risk is higher even if they have a mastectomy. Long-term survival, even in younger women, is similar whether the woman is treated with a breast-saving operation plus radiation or a total mastectomy. Total mastectomy, and sometimes bilateral mastectomy, is usually recommended in young women with a known or probable inherited risk for breast cancer as they are at substantially higher risk of developing cancer in the other breast.

What about sexuality, pregnancy, and fertility?

Many young women get diagnosed at a time when they are just about to start families and fertility may be a major concern. Treatments with chemotherapy may cause menopause (see Chapter 31). As soon as a young woman is diagnosed, fertility should be discussed as there may be options for storage of eggs or embryos prior to treatment, and this may provide an option for the future. There are fertility experts in most centres or to whom a woman can be referred. Pregnancy is not associated with an increase in breast cancer recurrence, but the women who had a pregnancy after breast cancer may not be representative of all women. As well, pregnancy may need to be delayed if there are treatments, in particular hormone treatments that need to be given over a long term (see Chapter 40).

Discuss these topics with your oncologist so a plan can be made that allows the optimal treatment for your breast cancer but also explores the options for future fertility. Each woman's situation needs to be considered on an individual basis.

Support groups

Some cancer centres have set up special support groups for young women with cancer as the psychological and sociological issues are different. Family and child-rearing issues may be important to juggle during treatment, and hearing from other women may be helpful. Job and economic issues often may cause significant anxieties. Relationships with partners, friends, and family have specific age-related features. There are also age-specific, web-based support groups that may be more appropriate for busy young women.

CHAPTER FORTY-TWO

Inherited breast cancer and genetic testing

Do my daughters have a higher risk of breast cancer?

THIS IS A FREQUENTLY ASKED QUESTION. At the outset, it is important to say that most daughters of women with breast cancer will not get breast cancer. However, because your daughters are female, this means that they live with at least the average risk of any woman. We also know that breast cancer can be passed on in families (see Chapter 3) so the question really becomes, "How much higher than the normal risk do my daughters face?"

To evaluate your daughter's risk of developing breast cancer, several points need to be considered:
- How many of your close relatives have breast cancer or ovarian cancer?
- How old were you when you developed breast cancer?
- Did the cancer affect one or both breasts?
- How old is your daughter?
- Does your daughter have any other risk factors?

Families with a strong history of breast cancer

Approximately 5 to 10% of breast cancers are due to an inherited genetic mutation. Two genes, BRCA1 and BRCA2, have already been identified as predisposing to a high risk of developing breast cancer. The mutations are mistakes on specific chromosomes that have been inherited either from the father or the mother. If a mutation is present, there is a high risk of developing cancer. In these families, relatives in three or more generations are often affected.

Genetic testing can be done to determine if you have inherited a mutation. Once the mutation is identified in someone who has already been diagnosed with breast cancer, the relatives of that person can be tested for that specific mutation. If you are identified as having the altered gene, the lifetime risk of developing breast cancer is 50 to 85% and there is also a higher chance of developing cancer in both breasts. The BRCA1 gene also confers a 40% lifetime risk of ovarian cancer. There is a small increased risk of prostate cancer in males who inherit the mutation. The BRCA2 gene confers an increased risk for both male and female breast cancer as well as ovarian cancer.

These cancers tend to occur 5 to 10 years earlier in each generation so it is important that planning and screening be undertaken early in the lives of women in these families. If an altered gene is identified in family members who have breast cancer, individuals who do not inherit the gene mutation have the same risk for breast cancer as the general population.

Not all hereditary breast cancers are caused by mutations in the BRCA1 and BRCA2 genes. Other genes such as CDH1, PTEN, STJ11, and TP53 have been shown to also increase the risk of developing breast cancer. Relatively uncommon genetic variants in genes such as CHEK2, ATM, NBS1, RAD51, BRIP1, and PALB2 are associated with a two-fold increase in the risk of breast cancer.

Your age at diagnosis

As women get older, the chance of developing breast cancer increases. This is unrelated to any special inherited tendency (see Chapter 2). Therefore, if the mother develops breast cancer at an older age, for example 75, the daughter's risk is only minimally higher. But if the mother developed cancer in her 30s, it is more likely that something genetic contributed to the cause of the cancer and that her daughter's risk is higher than normal.

Cancer of one or both breasts

If both breasts are affected, the chance of a genetic tendency toward breast cancer is higher. If cancer develops in both breasts in a woman younger than 50 years old, it indicates a substantially higher risk (5 to 10 times) in her daughters and also in the woman's sisters.

Number of family members with breast cancer

If three or more close blood relatives develop breast cancer or cancer of the ovary, it is more likely that some genetic error is being passed within the family, possibly associated with the BRCA1 or BRCA2 genes. This increases the risk of breast cancer developing in the daughter, son, sister, or brother of an affected woman. The members of the family may be either on the father's or mother's side. There is also a rare condition in which a gene called p53 is changed (mutated) and can be passed from a mother or father; this condition is associated with early breast cancer, brain cancers, and cancers known as sarcomas.

Genetic counselling and testing can estimate individual risk

If there is a very strong family history of breast cancer, an unaffected member of the family may be interested in genetic counselling to assess more accurately her individual risk of developing breast cancer. A strong family history is present when there are three or more cases of breast cancer in direct blood relatives, i.e., mother/daughter, aunt/niece, sister, grandmother, or a male member of the family. When there is a strong family history of breast cancer on the father's side, it can be passed on to the daughter even though the father did not develop cancer himself.

Certain ethnic groups or geographically defined populations have been found to have a high incidence of particular mutations in BRCA1, BRCA2, and some other genes. For instance, in the general population, 1 in every 800 individuals might have one of a wide variety of different mutations in BRCA1. In contrast, as many as 2 in every 100 Ashkenazi Jewish women have been shown to have one of just a few specific mutations. Another example is that a single mutation accounts for most of the cases of inherited breast cancer found in Iceland. These commonly occurring mutations in specific populations are called *founder mutations*. Founder mutations have been identified in many other ethnic groups or geographic populations (e.g., Sweden, French-Canadian, Dutch).

If you decide to have genetic counselling and testing, you will meet with a medical geneticist or genetic counsellor (or both), who will obtain a detailed family history. Your individual risk for breast cancer can be estimated and you will receive counselling regarding the pros, cons, and limitations of genetic testing for the abnormal mutation.

High-risk families: criteria for genetic risk assessment

Genetic testing may identify a mutation in an individual who is:
- A woman with breast cancer diagnosed at age 35 or younger OR
- A woman with ovarian cancer diagnosed at any age OR
- An Ashkenazi Jewish woman with breast or ovarian cancer diagnosed at any age
  OR a woman whose family history includes any *two* of the following:
- Breast cancer in two or more closely related family members (parents, siblings, children, grandparents, aunts, uncles)
- Cancers at an earlier age than expected in the general population (e.g., breast cancer before menopause, prostate cancer before age 50)
- Multiple primary cancers in different organs in one individual
- Cancers associated with known hereditary syndromes (e.g., breast/ovary, colon/uterus)

Before genetic testing is done, it is important to consider the implications of a positive or negative test, and the decisions you might make with such information. Genetic counselling provides an opportunity to discuss the limitations of genetic testing, how the results might affect you and your family's lives, and how you might use the test results. If you are interested in genetic counselling, have your doctor call your regional cancer centre to assess your eligibility and, if appropriate, the best way to make a referral.

Hereditary cancer programs

For women who carry an abnormal mutation for breast cancer such as the BRCA1 or BRCA2 genes, some cancer centres provide a high-risk clinic as part of a hereditary cancer program. In these clinics, women are monitored on a specific surveillance program in which screening and regular physical examinations play an important role in the early detection of cancer. Also, recent studies have shown that some medications may be capable of preventing breast cancer, e.g., tamoxifen (see Chapter 30). Medications may be prescribed for carefully assessed, high-risk individuals.

Screening and treatment recommendations

Screening of high risk women with identified or suspected mutations should include an annual mammogram after age 30. Recently, MRI scanning has been shown, in women with BRCA1 or BRCA2 mutations, to pick up earlier cancers that cannot be seen well on mammograms. Occasionally breast ultrasound may also be useful. It is recommended that high-risk women have a clinical breast examination every 6 months and a mammogram and MRI every 12 months. Screening ultrasounds may be used if MRI is not available or if abnormalities are found on other breast imaging examinations.

Some women at high risk choose to have bilateral mastectomy to decrease their risk of getting a cancer. Prophylactic mastectomy may decrease the risk of developing breast cancer by 98%. The risk of developing cancer is not eliminated 100% because at the time of mastectomy, a few breast glands may be left against the skin or chest wall muscles. Women who are planning to have a prophylactic mastectomy are encouraged to review breast reconstruction options including immediate reconstruction (see Chapter 34).

In most instances where there is a known BRCA1 or BRCA2 mutation, removal of the ovaries (oophorectomy) and fallopian tubes may be recommended after a woman has had her children. Removal of the ovaries and fallopian tubes decreases the risk of both ovarian cancer and breast cancer. Screening for ovarian cancer with a blood test called CA125, pelvic ultrasounds, and pelvic physical examination may not detect ovarian cancer in its early, curable stage.

Prophylactic surgery to decrease cancer risk is an option that needs careful discussion with the oncologist, surgeon, and genetic counsellor.

CHAPTER FORTY-THREE

Male breast cancer

MEN DEVELOP BREAST CANCER, but it is rare except in families with a BRCA2 gene mutation (see Chapter 42). The cancer usually appears as a lump under the nipple that often has been present for months but was ignored as the thought of it being breast cancer never entered the man's mind. A man with a new breast lump should have mammograms on both sides and a biopsy.

A male's likelihood of surviving breast cancer parallels that of a woman of the same age and stage of disease. Most men (90%) have ER-positive cancers. Treatment usually consists of mastectomy and sentinel node biopsy and, if necessary, an axillary dissection. Radiation may be added if the surgical margins are involved with cancer or if positive lymph nodes are found in the axilla. Tamoxifen, other hormone drugs, and/or chemotherapy are added with the same indications as have been described for a woman of the same age in Chapters 27 and 30. The side effects of treatment for breast cancer in men are much the same as described for women, but some hormone drugs may have different side effects related to differences in male hormones.

On a stage-for-stage basis men treated for breast cancer have an equal survival outcome as do women with breast cancer. However, since men typically present with breast cancer at a later stage than women, overall, men with breast cancer do not do quite as well as the average woman with breast cancer.

CHAPTER FORTY-FOUR

Complementary and alternative treatments

Complementary medicine REFERS TO TREATMENT that is used together with conventional medical treatment. *Alternative therapy* means treatment that is used in place of standard therapy. *Integrative medicine* is another term that refers to a practice that combines both conventional and complementary or alternative treatments for which there is evidence of safety and effectiveness.

What are complementary and alternative therapies?

"Alternative" and "complementary" are terms for a large number of health therapies that may be traditional treatments in a specific culture. Many of these treatments have value from the point of view of keeping hope alive and giving a woman a sense of control over her life again. However, most of these treatments have not been proven to reduce the chance that the cancer will regrow or to shrink cancers that have spread.

Complementary and alternative therapies include interventions from vitamins to diets, from relaxation and therapeutic touch to herbal remedies, from immune stimulants to metabolic therapy. It is not clear that all these therapies should be lumped into one category, but for the purposes of this chapter, it is useful to discuss their similarities.

It is estimated that over 60% of women with breast cancer use some form of complementary therapy. When vitamins, relaxation techniques, exercise, and visualization are included, the percentage of women using complementary or alternative therapies is much larger.

Why are complementary and alternative therapies described as "unproven"?

Most complementary and alternative therapies are referred to as unproven because they have not been subjected to rigorous scientific testing. Physicians depend on extensive experiments and studies to assess new therapies and evaluate their effectiveness and their toxicities. In contrast, the value of complementary or alternative therapies is often based on individual testimonials that the therapy was beneficial. This is not very dependable information because the particular circumstances and results cannot be confirmed. Many remedies have not been tested to see if the results can be reproduced in a consistent way. This is not to say that the treatments have no value, but most physicians feel uncomfortable placing their faith in a particular remedy without scientific facts to support its use. As well, without more information, it is impossible to know about potential side effects of such treatments—even herbal methods may have severe side effects. Much healing, however, occurs outside the realm of science.

Why do patients use complementary and alternative therapies?

Many women seek complementary and alternative therapies when they feel that their physicians predict only "doom and gloom." If the oncologist appears to have little to offer or if standard treatments offer only a small chance for cure, it is appealing to try something that seems hopeful and positive. As well, many of the practitioners of holistic approaches are very charismatic and optimistic. Who wouldn't seek the reassurance of a practitioner who gives hope rather than one who seems more negative?

Many women also adopt complementary treatments because they feel empowered in choosing and directing their own care. This is a very positive attitude that helps one's psychological health during the ordeal of cancer therapy. This assertiveness shouldn't be restricted to choosing methods of complementary therapy. Each patient should participate in the decisions regarding her conventional treatment: the type of surgery, radiation, chemotherapy, and hormones.

Not only does a woman often feel powerless, but so do many friends and family members, who sometimes steer women toward alternative treatments because they want to help. Other women simply have a general mistrust of the conventional medical establishment.

Complementary or alternative therapies are often promoted as less toxic and more natural, with claims of boosting the immune system to attack the cancer in a natural way. Many claim that holistic programs are gentler, less invasive, and more individualized. However, you must be aware that side effects can still occur, and these treatments are complementary or alternative because they have not been proven to have an effect on cancer progression, even though there may be a seemingly rational logic to their recommendation.

Any treatment plan should be considered in terms of the goals of the treatment, the duration of the therapy, the side effects, and the alternatives. The same questions should be asked of complementary and alternative therapies and standard therapy practitioners. All health care providers should be able to address these questions.

Types of complementary and alternative therapies

The most common complementary cancer therapies can be categorized into the following groups: biologically based/natural products, mind/body medicine, manipulative and body-based practices, energy therapies, whole medicine systems, and others.

Biologically based/natural products

This is a large area and includes herbal medicines (known as botanicals), vitamins, minerals, other "natural products," and "biological" therapies. Some of these treatments are dietary supplements that may or may not be helpful. There is some evidence that high doses of water-soluble vitamins can be toxic and that other vitamins may interfere with standard therapies such as chemotherapy. Antioxidants have been shown to have potential interference with both chemotherapy and radiation, and a review of the literature suggested that caution should be used when taking antioxidants during standard therapy. There have been concerns that some natural health products may be contaminated by fungi and that some can cause liver damage. Many natural products may also interfere with the other medications that many women take and therefore it is important to tell your doctor if you are considering taking natural products during your standard cancer therapy. Some of the biological treatments have been shown to increase the risk of bleeding due to interference with the production of platelets, which are important in blood clotting. Many vitamins have been studied; beta carotene was rigorously studied in lung cancer, with surprising and disappointing results as there was a suggestion of a worse outcome for those persons on high doses of beta carotene.

There is hope that some diets may be important in preventing breast cancer and also preventing breast cancer recurrence. It is not clear which diet is the best, but it appears that not gaining weight after a diagnosis of breast cancer, obtaining and maintaining a normal body mass index (BMI), and watching overall caloric intake is important (see Chapter 35). There is no evidence that a particular diet can prevent cancer, but there have been suggestions that lower fat and lower calorie diets may reduce the risk of recurrence. The emphasis is on maintaining a normal BMI, which may involve losing weight. Common sense and the Canada Health Food Guide appear appropriate. See Chapter 35 for more information on diet, nutrition, and BMI.

Many traditional herbalists, particularly from traditional Chinese medicine, recommend a variety of herbal remedies to promote both health and decrease breast cancer recurrence. Most of these therapies have not been rigorously studied. Some contain estrogen supplements, which should be used with caution in women with estrogen-sensitive breast cancer. It may be worthwhile ensuring that your herbalist is a member of an association that has credentials and that he or she has received appropriate training. There are websites that provide guidance to Canadian patients on this issue (www.camline.ca). Natural health products are now regulated by Health Canada. In many provinces in Canada naturopathic physicians and traditional medicine practitioners are regulated and it is worthwhile ensuring that when buying products you check they meet approved standards. Some people may sell products they bring into the country that are sold outside these guidelines and it is worthwhile to know this prior to purchasing.

Immune therapies are considered biologic treatments and depend on the theory that cancer is due to an immune defect. The theory is that if the immune system can be strengthened, then the cancer can be controlled. The immune system is a very complex and poorly understood part of our make-up. Although some cancers do seem to be directly related to deficiencies in the immune system, others occur without any apparent connection to the immune system. Researchers and immunologists are struggling to determine what role the immune system has in the treatment of various cancers. At this time, despite years of research, there are many unanswered questions. Vaccines and medications to boost the immune system have validity for some cancers. There are many vaccines being studied in clinical trials, but at this time there is no evidence that an overall immune stimulation is beneficial against breast cancer.

Mind/body medicine

Mind/body practices focus on the interaction among the brain, mind, body, and behaviour with the intent of using the mind to affect physical functioning and to improve health. The therapies used include meditation, exercise such as yoga, breathing techniques, hypnotherapy, tai chi, and relaxation exercises. Many of these practices are used in traditional healing and may be helpful in promoting relaxation, decreased stress, and improved quality of life.

Acupuncture may also be included in this group, although it is also considered a component of energy medicine, manipulative and body-based practices, and also Chinese medicine. Acupuncture has been shown to be helpful for pain control and in palliative care.

Many of these practices are being studied in clinical trials to assess their role in specific areas of treatment. As well, for many women these practices may be lifestyle changes that promote health and a sense of empowerment at a time when this has been severely affected.

Manipulative and body-based practices

These practices focus on the structures and systems of the body with the belief that improving these aspects of the body, including the bones, joints, lymphatic and circulatory systems, and the soft tissues will promote healing and health. Chiropractors, massage, physical therapists, and osteopaths work on the spinal system, which is included in this aspect of complementary and alternative therapies. There are a number of techniques that may be employed. Chiropractors may do manipulation. Massage therapists may work on tissues through massage, and physical therapists may do a combination of treatments. These therapies may relieve pain, induce relaxation, reduce anxiety and stress, and improve quality of life. For specific areas of the body these treatments may be very helpful. Their effect on reducing cancer risk has not been proven but certainly manipulative and body-based practices have been used for hundreds of years.

Energy medicine

Energy medicine includes many forms of therapy including acupuncture (as mentioned above in the mind/body section), reiki, qi gong, therapeutic and healing touch, as well as magnet or light therapy. Some of the practices are based on harnessing energy fields or biofields to affect health. Others are more subtle and are thought to engage energy that we have inside us as human beings. These include qi gong and healing touch. The concept of visual imagery is that mental energy can be focused through visualization to destroy cancer cells or stop their growth. These therapies have not been proven to have an effect on cancer growth on their own but they promote one's sense of responsibility and control in a way that can act with other healing remedies. Anecdotally, healing touch, when provided by a good practitioner, may be helpful for pain and nausea.

Whole medical systems

Some complementary or alternative practitioners provide "whole medical systems" interventions, which are supposed to deal with unique healing systems that will both reduce cancer risk and promote overall health. These systems include traditional Chinese medicine, naturopathic medicine, or others such as Ayruvedic medicine. Many of these combine naturopathic treatments with mind/body, manipulative, and energy medicine. As well, standard chemotherapy may be included in the treatment in some centres that provide whole medical systems. Others shun standard therapy in favour of the use of their system exclusively. There are no scientific studies to support these approaches.

What are the risks of these treatments?

The risks of complementary and alternative therapies are related to the lack of scientific testing. We depend on regulations to keep our food safe. We test and categorize which additives are approved, and legally require that they be listed on the box or package to protect us as consumers. These safeguards exist for alternative cancer treatments that are regulated by Health Canada and other agencies, although some practitioners import their own products that are not included in these safeguards. As well, the costs can be prohibitive. A therapy that promises a cure makes people with cancer susceptible to paying potentially large amounts of money for something with no firm evidence of benefit.

The practitioners of alternative treatments may be very ethical and well-meaning, and there are now websites that attempt to protect patients from quacks and crooks who are also in the business.

Another problem is that if the cancer does not respond to a change in, say, behaviour or diet, the patient may feel like a failure. Many people already (mistakenly) feel responsible for getting cancer in the first place—due to their diet, stress, or other lifestyle factors in their past. Although accepting responsibility for making treatment choices is worthwhile, blaming oneself can be very damaging.

Finally, some cancers are very treatable and can be cured with standard therapy. Although every patient should have a choice of treatment, there are concerns that if a curative treatment is rejected in favour of an alternative therapy the chance of being cured may be lost because of a delay in initiating anti-cancer treatment of proven benefit.

Ongoing studies of complementary and alternative therapies may provide the information necessary to properly assess and recommend various treatments. We eagerly await the results.

Open discussion builds trust

Many patients are hesitant to discuss their interest in complementary or alternative therapies with their doctors. However, it is important that the physician be informed for the benefit of both the patient and the doctor.

Patients who opt for complementary or alternative treatments should not be hesitant to maintain contact and receive treatment from their conventional doctors or to return to them when the time seems right.

Additional information

The Canadian Cancer Society produced a booklet about complementary and alternative therapies in 2009. A downloadable PDF in English or French is available from their website (www. cancer.ca). It is easiest to find if you search the alphabetical listing of their publications.

CHAPTER FORTY-FIVE

Clinical research:
Looking for better answers

Why are clinical studies important?

AS MOST WOMEN QUICKLY LEARN, there are a lot of unanswered questions about breast cancer. What is/are the cause(s)? Can we prevent it? What new treatment or approach might give better results than we're getting right now? Is there some way of curing breast cancer permanently?

Research is about improving care. Research studies (also called *trials*) try to answer questions about how to improve care. It's an ongoing process, with questions constantly being asked, and researchers continually looking for better ways of treating patients. Sometimes we forget that the treatments we now consider as "standard" for breast cancer (drugs, surgery, radiation) were at one time considered experimental. It is because women with breast cancer have volunteered to participate in research studies that the current treatments are available.

What are the steps in testing a new treatment?

All potential treatments go through the same type of rigorous evaluation process that can be illustrated with the example of the testing of a new drug.

All new drug treatments begin in the laboratory. If extensive tests in test tubes and mice suggest that a new drug has potential in treating breast cancer, it is tested in humans in a preliminary (phase 1) study to check side effects and to establish a dose level at which side effects are acceptable. The safe dose level is then tested in a small group of women to determine its effect in controlling the cancer (phase 2). In this phase the question is, "Does the drug work at a dose that is safe in humans?" Phase 1 and 2 studies usually involve volunteers with advanced or metastatic breast cancer.

If the results are still promising, the question then arises whether the new drug is better than the standard treatment. To determine this, a third (phase 3) study is done in which volunteers are randomly selected to receive either the new drug or the old (current standard) treatment. If it is not known which treatment is superior, it is ethical to compare the treatments in consenting, volunteer women with breast cancer.

Scientific studies such as these must follow rigid statistical rules to confirm that the information gained is reliable and valid. It is also important that patients give their consent before they are included in any study. The issues of ethical conduct and scientific rigor of a study are reviewed and must be approved by an institutional research ethics board before a research study may begin enrolling subjects.

Other treatments can be tested in a similar fashion. For example, ongoing studies are evaluating the role of partial breast radiation as compared to whole breast radiation, the need for axillary dissection if a sentinel lymph node is positive, the optimum duration of hormonal therapy, and the role of an anti-diabetes medication to prevent recurrence of breast cancer.

Media reports about advances in understanding cancer or new treatments are often based on very preliminary data. Sometimes, a promising phase 2 study or even an animal study may be reported as a "clinical" breakthrough. This is confusing for the public and physicians as well. Until a new treatment can be confirmed to be both effective and superior to standard therapy in large studies, it cannot be recommended as the new standard of care. However, with persistence and with the participation of patient volunteers, new therapies are being introduced every year.

What should I do if I'm asked to be part of a study?

Participation in any study is voluntary. If you are asked to consider enrolling in a study, you should understand why the study is being done, what is already known of the treatment's side effects and benefits, and about any alternative treatment options. Many phase 2 and phase 3 trials use treatments that have been available for some time, so there could be considerable information available. On the other hand, it is important to understand that the primary aim of a phase 1 trial is to define the side effects of a novel treatment, since usually very few patients have received this treatment.

Before any study is done, hospital ethics committees evaluate the research plan to ensure that the rights of the patient are protected and that the study is ethical in its design and implementation. These ethics committees always include members of the lay public. Written, informed consent must be obtained from each patient before they participate in a research study. This means that the researcher must carefully discuss the study with each potential participant, explaining the reasons for it, the risks and benefits, other options the patient has in terms of treatment, and that study participation is voluntary. Some research studies require the patient to have extra blood or imaging studies—often at no cost to the patient, or to have extra follow-up visits at the cancer centre. The patient should not sign consent to participate unless she has had all her questions answered thoroughly.

Ultimately, each woman is free to decide what is in her best interest, and must be comfortable in choosing whether to take part in a study. Also, she must understand that she may elect to subsequently withdraw her consent for study participation. It is through the commitment of thousands of women participating in clinical research that many advances have been made in the treatment of breast cancer, and the authors of this book encourage you to consider participation in a clinical research study if one is available to you.

CHAPTER FORTY-SIX

Awareness and advocacy

Contributed by Judith Caldwell, breast cancer survivor and Founder of the Canadian Breast Cancer Foundation – BC/Yukon Chapter

THE GOOD NEWS IS that most of us live after an encounter with breast cancer. The tough news is that we still can't expect everyone to be cured and we can't reassure our daughters that breast cancer is preventable. When I was in high school, my friend Cathy's mum developed breast cancer and had radical surgery. Thankfully, surgical techniques have improved, and today the type of surgery she endured has almost totally disappeared. We knew that one side of her body was disfigured, that the arm on her affected side was swollen and painful, and that she was very, very sick. We whispered about it behind Cathy's back, but never asked her how everything was at home. We weren't heartless, only young, frightened, embarrassed, and unable to find the right words. In retrospect, I realize that we figured that if we denied that the life of one of our favourite mums was being threatened, that breast cancer would go away and leave us, and our own mums, unscathed.

Decades later, with close to two decades of survival under my belt, I know that silence and denial kill. Our job as advocates is to break the silence and focus an uncompromising light on all the issues surrounding breast cancer.

The physical, emotional, and financial effects of this disease can be devastating. While each of us experiences breast cancer differently, most of us ride a roller coaster of overwhelming anxiety, grief, sadness, anger, frustration, hope, denial, black humour, and the fear of a truncated future.

On our bodies, there's an indelible physical reminder that our lives have been put in peril, and that breast cancer may return to threaten our lives once again, and perhaps kill us. Advocacy offers a means to channel our energies and to do something positive about a situation over which we still have no means of prevention and precious little control. It's a way to save lives and to forge purpose out of an apparently chaotic, senseless situation.

Most of us who develop breast cancer are taken by surprise, with no family history or obvious risk factors. We face an instant medical crash course in learning enough about the disease to make critical treatment choices. Usually, it's not until the immediate crises of diagnosis and treatment decisions have passed that an awareness of the staggering scope of breast cancer becomes apparent. When the huge number of women affected becomes apparent, a "Why me?" cry turns into a "why not me?" realization.

With breast cancer we confront the uncomfortable issue of breasts and the values of femininity, sexuality, and nurturing we have placed upon them. We relish memories of babies nursing at our breasts, lovers' caresses, and holding those we cherish in a soft embrace. On every newsstand, in every movie and TV show, we are swamped with images exploiting cleavage, with never-ending expectations of how a woman must look to be womanly. It is essential to get rid of any embarrassment you might have over having breast cancer. The public needs to know that treating breast cancer is about saving lives, and that even with changed bodies, life, love, sex, and femininity carry on. Indeed, a re-evaluation of priorities and values in the shadow of breast cancer may yield a more conscious appreciation of life. Believe me, no one signs on for cancer to have a "growth experience," but it often happens.

Advocacy comes in many forms. We need to corner the politicians who control health care and research purse strings to determine how much money has been targeted for breast cancer and how it is being spent. Charitable organizations should be questioned on their spending priorities. We need to know how recent research has benefited patients in screening centres, clinics, and hospitals. We need to understand the financial burden that hits a family when breast cancer causes a woman to leave the workplace.

Breast cancer has been around for centuries and has received a great deal of attention over the past decades. So, why does it remain a hot, public topic? Is it because our aging population, with active, educated, influential women with huge responsibilities at home and at work, is edging into the most susceptible age bracket? Is it because sexual issues are more in the open? Is it because of the continuing public awareness that more money is still needed for breast cancer research, education, and swift treatment? Is it due to the pointed questions about why there hasn't been more progress in finding preventive strategies and cures, even though the media tout cancer cure breakthroughs on a regular basis?

It is also our job to inform women of the realities of breast cancer and to encourage them to take realistic care of themselves. It is true that thousands of Canadian women have had their futures stolen from them and die prematurely every year of the disease. It is also true that over three million North American women are living with a previous diagnosis of breast cancer and are hoping that it never returns.

It is tragic that too many women in their most vulnerable years, 50 and over, are not yet using the mammogram programs available to them. The age for beginning screening is no longer controversial. Although it's not yet a 100% perfect early detection system, I am grateful, as are so many other women, that my tumour was found in my mid-40s, earlier than it would otherwise have been without this technology. Without it, my tumour would have remained an undetected time bomb in my body for months or years, and I would likely have been faced with much more difficult treatment.

Across North America, information is not easily available in the languages of smaller cultural groups. Not all women know how to perform breast self-examination or to recognize changes in their breasts. Not all women know that, if they are diagnosed, there are treatment options and that the earlier the diagnosis, the better the options will be. Not all women realize that their doctors are there to serve them and that they have rights to full information, their own personal medical records, second opinions, and choices. Not all families know that genetic screening clinics are available to give excellent information on the potential susceptibility of women whose families included generations of women who were previously affected by the disease. Our moral support and willingness to accompany others through the maze of new, complex information and difficult choices is a front-line form of advocacy.

The most basic tools of advocacy are information, facts, figures, and a clear understanding of the social and financial impact of the disease. However, the full breast cancer story cannot be told highlighting finances and statistics alone. The personal is political, and stories of women and families facing breast cancer must be told. The pain of lost battles must be made real and the hope that comes from the lives of long-time survivors spread. As advocates, we must recognize that influence is created and decisions are based on gut reactions as well as logic.

So, what can only one person do?

- Educate yourself before you do anything. Learn as much as you can about the disease and the issues that interest you. For example, if funding is your concern, find out how funds are being spent by reading annual reports of groups raising money. Find out how much money is being spent on administration and how much is going directly to further the cause. Apply to be part of grant-allocation committees. Ask for a report card on previous grants. What has been learned? Or, as another example, if long waiting lists are your issue, ensure you get the correct, current statistics. Incorrect information will weaken your effectiveness.
- Focus. Advocacy comes in many forms: support groups, fund raising, education, raising concerns about genetic testing, political lobbying, and ensuring mammography clinics have the best equipment. Keep your goals clear. Be bold in asking people with the skills you need to help you.
- Find others. Place an ad in the local newspaper asking for others interested in the cause to contact you. Host a meeting. Many an influential group has first started around a kitchen table. Create a website and link to other groups through social media. Buddies help. As one of the founding paddlers of Abreast in a Boat, the first internationally competitive dragon boat team entirely powered by breast cancer survivors, I know that personal support and public advocacy are close kin. One can power the other. What started

out in Canada with 24 women paddlers in one experimental boat has morphed into over 150 crews world wide, from Canada to Poland, from Singapore to New Zealand. These teams won't be ignored and the numbers of paddlers in the dragon boats are dwarfed by the thousands of aware supporters cheering their efforts and becoming educated about the numbers of people affected by the disease.

- Amplify your voice with social media. Today's advocates need to know how to network using social media effectively. A social network is an online community of people who share interests, in this case, breast cancer issues. Social media has the power to facilitate conversations across continents and to galvanize audiences around breast cancer topics. New networking and information tools will inevitably emerge and old ones will change, but currently we have powerful tools including, but not limited to: Facebook, Twitter, Winks, YouTube, social bookmarking (e.g., Delicious), email, podcasting, and blogging. These can bring like-minded people together in different ways. For example, the right tool at the right time can educate, encourage people to interact and discuss issues, gather people together, demonstrate procedures, and even put you on world-wide video. Imagine the influence of broadcasting your voice through podcasting, sharing your photos with Flickr, posting videos to YouTube, and sharing informative websites through bookmarking. How powerful could it be to connect with content experts worldwide by reading their blogs and by creating your own blog for others to access? Advocates must be up-to-date. RSS feeds and Delicious web profiles can put vital news sources literally in your hand. If you don't know how to use these Internet tools, find someone who does. Like any physical tool, the forms of social media may be used inappropriately and carry inaccurate information. It's up to the users to verify content and use the tools judiciously.
- Network strategically. Consider joining your group with other breast cancer groups locally, provincially, nationally, and internationally. A broader base and co-operative, strategic alignments with similar breast cancer organizations can give you more influence with governments. After

all, governments can alter directions and implement new health policies. Creating good relations with the government in power and the opposition parties will be vital for your success. Consider cross-marketing and co-operative events. Through the web, learn from the success of other advocacy organizations whether concerned with breast cancer or other issues.

- Make friends with the media and make it easy for the media to follow your progress. Look for photo opportunities and take pictures of events. Write brief personal interest stories. Cultivate specific TV, radio, and print contacts and educate them on your cause with concise, factual information sheets. Find a credible spokesperson.

- Speak out courageously in public, especially at election time. This is the time to hold their feet to the fire. Ask each political party the same, specific, tough questions you want answered. Compare their answers. For example, how would each party deal with long hospital and surgical waiting lists? Will they fund new drug therapies?

The job of finding the cause(s) and ways to prevent breast cancer is a team effort, resembling a marathon more than a sprint. Our researchers, nurses, clinicians, and everyone else on our medical teams are people with families and financial obligations like the rest of us. Their skills are being sought internationally. Like it or not, we have to compete for their expertise. We need to continue to attract sustained, secure funding and to convince our governments and charitable organizations to set priorities. What could be more important than putting corporate donations and tax dollars to work to save bodies and lives?

Even if we had a magic bullet, a magic cure for all forms of breast cancer right now, we would still have to treat women currently diagnosed and we would have to scour the country to find others who have the disease hidden in their bodies. So, we need a prevention strategy. In advocating for breast cancer we need determined optimism and courage. Take heart, courage is contagious.

Breast self-examination technique

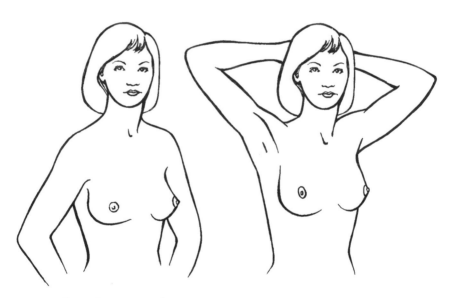

Standing, arms down,
to check basic appearance.

Raising arms
to look for changes.

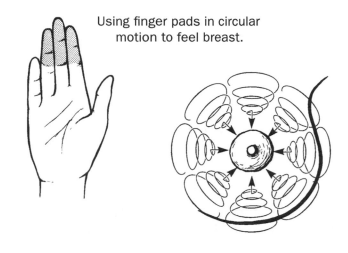

Using finger pads in circular motion to feel breast.

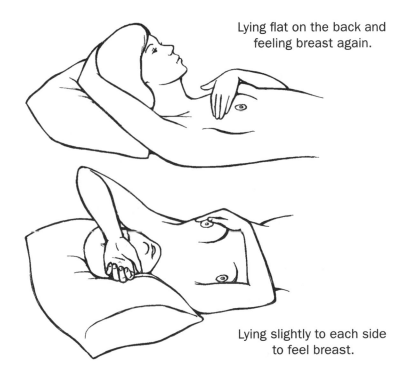

Lying flat on the back and feeling breast again.

Lying slightly to each side to feel breast.

Glossary

Adjuvant therapy: Treatment that is given in addition to the initial, apparently complete surgery to help prevent the cancer from recurring. Often called "insurance" against recurrence of cancer. Adjuvant therapy is given after surgery, whereas neoadjuvant therapy is given prior to surgery (see neoadjuvant therapy).

Androgen: Male hormone that may be used as a drug to treat breast cancer.

Angiogenesis: Literally "new blood vessel growth" from the Greek *angio* (vessel) and *genesis* (birth or growth). Angiogenesis is a required part of cancer growth because the new blood vessels are necessary to bring a supply of oxygen and nutrients to the cancer cells.

Angiosarcoma: A rare type of cancer that develops from the cells of the blood vessels. It occurs in approximately 1 of every 1,000 women who receive radiation therapy after mastectomy or breast conserving surgery.

Aromatase: An enzyme located in the fat and other body tissues that is involved in the production of estrogen from other steroid hormones, in postmenopausal women.

Aromatase inhibitors: Drugs that can block the action of the aromatase enzyme. This block decreases the production of estrogen in postmenopausal women. These drugs are used as hormone treatments in postmenopausal women with tumours that are estrogen receptor positive. Common aromatase inhibitors are anastrozole (Arimidex), letrozole (Femara), and exemestane (Aromasin).

Atypical cells: Cells that appear abnormal but not frankly cancerous when viewed under the microscope.

Axilla: The underarm area between the armpit and the collarbone.

Benign tumour: A harmless tumour that is not cancerous.

Biopsy: A procedure in which a small piece of tissue is removed to be studied under the microscope to help make a diagnosis. A biopsy may be done using surgery (an open biopsy) or with a fine or core needle inserted in the doctor's office or using ultrasound or mammographic guidance.

Brachytherapy: The use of catheters or radioactive pellets directly inserted into the breast to deliver radiation internally to the tissue surrounding the tumour or surgical cavity.

Breast implant: A round or teardrop-shaped sac filled with salt water or silicone that is placed under the skin and muscle of the chest wall after mastectomy to create a breast shape or improve the shape of an existing breast.

Breast prosthesis: An artificial breast form that can be worn externally to replace the breast shape after a mastectomy.

Breast reconstruction: Surgical procedures (several types) that create a breast shape with or without a nipple after breast surgery for cancer. This may involve insertion of a breast implant or creation of a breast shape from other body tissues.

Calcifications: Tiny deposits of calcium that may signify cancer and can be seen on a mammogram.

Carcinoma: Another word for cancer.

Cancer: The abnormal and uncontrolled growth of cells that may invade and destroy surrounding tissues.

Capsular contracture: Scar tissue that may form after an implant reconstruction that makes the implant hard and rounded.

Chemotherapy: Treatment for cancer involving the use of drugs.

Circulating cells: Free floating cancer cells found in a blood sample.

Clinical trial: A research study designed to test a new therapy or treatment approach.

Complementary therapy: Interventions used together with traditional medicine but which have not been proven to have a direct anti-cancer effect.

Cyst: A non-cancerous sac or lump filled with fluid.

Dissection: Surgical cutting open of a part of the body.

Duct ectasia: Widened (or dilated) milk ducts.

Ductal carcinoma in situ (DCIS): Cancer that is confined within the milk ducts; no invasion.

Edema: Swelling of body tissue due to accumulation of fluid. This may occur in the arm or breast after removal of lymph nodes during treatment for breast cancer.

Estrogen: A sex hormone that is responsible for the development of female characteristics such as breasts and broadening of the hips at the time of puberty. Estrogen has a key role in the menstrual cycle and pregnancy and stimulates the growth of some breast cancers. It is made in the ovaries before menopause and to a lesser extent, throughout the body fat after menopause.

Estrogen receptor (ER): A protein in the cancer cell that binds to the hormone estrogen. A cancer cell that is estrogen receptor-rich (or positive) is usually sensitive to hormones.

Fat necrosis: A lump of dead fat cells in the breast that is often tender and may occur after an injury severe enough to cause bruising such as a car accident, physical abuse, or breast surgery.

Fibroadenoma: A firm, round, fibrous lump, most often found in young women and which does not turn cancerous.

Fine needle aspiration biopsy: A biopsy technique in which a thin needle is inserted into the body and a few cells or some fluid is removed for diagnosis.

Fine wire localization: A technique to direct a surgical biopsy to an area of the breast which is abnormal on a mammogram but which cannot be felt. A thin wire is placed into the breast under ultrasound or mammographic control to guide the surgeon to the correct part of the breast.

Founder mutations: A commonly occurring genetic mutation in a specific population; it results in a high risk of developing cancer.

HER2: A cancer gene (oncogene) that is overexpressed (makes too much HER2 protein). Found in approximately 20% of breast cancers. This oncogene may cause the cancer to be more aggressive. Also called the Her2/neu gene.

Herceptin: The trade name of trastuzamab, an anti-HER2 antibody that is useful in controlling some breast cancers that overexpress HER2 (see HER2).

Hormone receptors: Proteins in cancer (and other) cells that bind to hormones such as estrogen (estrogen receptors; ER) or progesterone (progesterone receptor; PR). The binding of the hormone to the receptor causes a biological response in the cell, e.g., to stimulate the cell to grow.

Hormone therapy: Treatment for breast cancer that involves altering the hormone levels in the body. This may involve removing the ovaries or the use of specific drugs given as tablets or injections.

Hormones: Normally occurring chemicals produced by specific parts of the body (glands) that travel through the blood stream to another location in the body where they cause a change in a structure or function of a body tissue (e.g., estrogen in young women is produced in the ovaries and causes the breasts to develop).

Hyperplasia: Cells that divide and accumulate in excessive numbers but are not yet cancerous.

In situ breast cancer: Cancer growing within the milk ducts or milk glands of the breast.

Invasive cancer: Cancer that has extended or spread out of the milk ducts to invade adjacent tissues or organs.

LHRH-agonists: A class of hormone therapy that works by interfering with the normal control of ovarian function in premenopausal women.

Lobules (lobular): That part of the breast housing the milk glands.

Locally advanced cancer: Breast cancer that is very large, growing into the skin, or spread to many axillary lymph nodes. Usually treated with hormones, chemotherapy, and radiation prior to surgery.

Lumpectomy: A surgical procedure in which the tumour and a small margin of surrounding normal breast tissue is removed. Lumpectomy may also be called a *partial mastectomy, segmental mastectomy, wide excision,* or *breast conserving surgery.*

Lymph nodes: Small lima bean-shaped structures grouped at various locations along the lymph system in the body (e.g., armpits, neck, groin). They act as the main "filters" to defend against infections and can be a site for cancer to spread. Lymph nodes under the arm are frequently removed as part of breast cancer surgery to determine if cancer has spread beyond the breast.

Lymphatic system: The network of vessels throughout the body that carries lymph fluid to and from all the tissues of the body.

Lymphedema: See Edema.

Magnetic Resonance Imaging (MRI): A body scan using strong magnetic fields to examine internal body structures.

Malignant tumour: A cancerous lump that is harmful because it grows out of control and invades and destroys surrounding tissues and can spread to other parts of the body (metastasize).

Mammogram: An X-ray of the breast.

Mastectomy: A surgical procedure in which the whole breast is removed. May be a called total, modified-radical, radical, simple, or subcutaneous mastectomy. For partial mastectomy see Lumpectomy.

Menopause: The time of life when a woman's monthly periods stop because her ovaries have stopped making estrogen.

Metastases: The spread of a cancer from one organ where growth started, to another part of the body (also as a verb —to metastasize).

Microcalcifications: Very tiny calcifications.

Mutation: An alteration in a gene that causes the gene to function abnormally.

Neoadjuvant therapy: Radiation, chemotherapy, or hormonal therapy given prior to surgery to enhance the effect of surgery or to make the surgery easier. Neoadjuvant therapy is given prior to surgery, whereas adjuvant therapy is given after surgery.

Necrosis: The death of cells.

Oncologist: A physician who specializes in the treatment of patients with cancer.

Palpation: Examination with the hands; to feel.

Papillomas: Small growths inside the milk duct that are benign, but may cause bleeding from the nipple.

Partial breast radiation: A technique to deliver radiation to just the quarter of the breast thought to be most at risk of cancer recurrence.

Pathologist: A physician who specializes in the diagnosis of disease by studying the structure and function of normal and abnormal cells and tissues of the body.

Phylloides tumour: An uncommon type of breast cancer that arises from the fibrous tissue rather than the milk ducts in the breast.

Phytoestrogens: Weak, estrogen-like compounds found in foods such as soybeans and flaxseeds.

Predictive factor: A test of cancer characteristic (e.g., estrogen receptor or HER2 status) that predicts the likelihood that a cancer will respond to a particular treatment (e.g., estrogen receptor status predicts response to hormone therapy; HER2 status predicts response to the drug Herceptin).

Primary cancer: A cancer in the organ of origin.

Progesterone: A female sex hormone involved in a number of functions, including the menstrual cycle and pregnancy.

Progesterone receptor (PR): A protein in the cancer cell that, together with the ER status, indicates the likelihood that a breast cancer will respond to a hormone.

Prognosis: An estimate of the expected course of the disease.

Prognostic factor: A test or cancer characteristic (e.g., size of the tumour, grade or number of lymph nodes involved) that indicates the likelihood of future cancer regrowth.

Prophylactic: A preventive treatment that may involve any type of therapy, e.g., drugs, surgery, radiation.

Prosthesis: An artificial device that is attached to the body to substitute for a part of the body that is missing.

Radiation pneumonitis: Inflammation and scarring of the lung that may cause cough or shortness of breath several months after radiation therapy if a large amount of the lung is treated.

Radiotherapy (radiation therapy, RT): The use of high-energy radiation for the treatment of cancer.

Recurrence: The reappearance or regrowth of cancer. The recurrence may be in the original site (a local recurrence), in the adjacent lymph nodes (a regional recurrence), or elsewhere in the body (a systemic or distant recurrence).

Remission: When there is no detectable evidence of cancer on physical examination or with medical tests.

Risk factor: Something that increases the chance of getting a disease. A risk factor may be either acquired from the environment or inherited.

Sarcoma: A type of cancer arising from the connecting tissues of the body (e.g., the muscles, bones, nerves, fatty tissues).

Sclerosing adenosis: Scarring and inflammation around the breast glands that may show up as fine calcifications on a mammogram.

Screening: Tests done on a well person to detect unsuspected disease.

Secondary cancer: A cancer that has spread to another site. Also called *metastatic cancer.*

Sentinel node: The lymph node closest to or receiving the first lymph drainage from the breast, usually in the axilla (armpit).

Sentinel node biopsy: A technique to identify the lymph node most likely to be involved if cancer has spread outside the breast. It involves injecting blue dye and/or a radio-active tracer around the tumour and tracing the lymph flow to the nearest (or sentinel) lymph node.

Staging: The clinical examinations and tests done at the time of diagnosis to determine the extent of the cancer in the body.

Subcutaneous: The area immediately below the skin.

Sutures: Stitches used to close up a surgical wound.

Systemic: Affecting the body in general rather than one specific part.

Tamoxifen: An anti-estrogen drug and the most widely used hormone therapy to treat breast cancer metastases and/or help prevent the recurrence of breast cancer.

Telangiectasia: Small, spidery, prominent blood vessels that may appear on the skin 18 to 24 months after radiation therapy.

Tumour: Any abnormal growth of tissue. Can be cancerous (malignant) or non-cancerous (benign).

White blood cells: Cells in the blood stream that detect and fight infection, foreign material, and abnormal cells.

Additional reading

General information

100 questions and answers about breast cancer. 2nd ed. Brown, Zora K; Freeman, Harold P; Platt, Elizabeth. Boston: Jones and Bartlett Publishers, 2007. (book)

Abreast and the Rest. BC/Yukon Women's Cancer Alliance. www.abreastandtherest.ca (quarterly newsletter)

Companion and reference guide for women with breast cancer. Quarry Integrated Communications; Gelmon, Karen A. Mississauga: Hoffmann-La Roche, 2009. (book)

Healthy eating and fitness

American Cancer Society complete guide to nutrition for cancer survivors: eating well, staying well during and after cancer, 2nd ed. Grant, Barbara L; American Cancer Society. Atlanta: American Cancer Society, 2010. (book)

Eating well when you have cancer: a guide to good nutrition. Canadian Cancer Society. Toronto: Canadian Cancer Society, 2008. (44 page booklet)

Exercise for health: an exercise guide for breast cancer survivors. Vallance, Jeff; Courneya, Kerry S. Edmonton: Athabasca University, University of Alberta, 2008. (book)

Exercises after breast surgery: a guide for women. Canadian Cancer Society. Toronto: Canadian Cancer Society, 2006. (24 page booklet)

Goes down easy: recipes to help you cope with the challenge of eating during cancer treatment. Mecklinger, Elise. Toronto: Princess Margaret Hospital Foundation, 2006. (book)

Nutrition guide for women with breast cancer. Developed by the BC Cancer Agency, Oncology Nutrition and HealthLink BC, 2010. (69 page booklet)

Reconstruction

100 questions and answers about breast surgery. Disa, Joseph J; Kuechel, Marie Czenko. Sudbury: Jones and Bartlett Publishers, 2006. (book)

Breast reconstruction guidebook: issues and answers from research to recovery. Steligo, Kathy. San Carlos, CA: Carlo Press, 2003. (book)

Breast reconstruction using the TRAM flap. Bowman, Cameron. Vancouver: Banford Communications, 2003. (DVD)

Reconstructing Aphrodite. Lorant, Terry; Eskenazi, Loren; Hayse, Helga. Burlington, VT: Verve Editions, 2001. (book)

Understanding breast reconstruction surgery: is it for me? BC Cancer Agency Breast Tumour Group; Lennox, Peter. Vancouver: BC Cancer Agency Multi-Media Services, 2007. (DVD)

Complementary and alternative therapy

American Cancer Society complete guide to complementary and alternative cancer methods. 2nd ed. Ades, Terri; Russell, Jill; Rovere, Amy; American Cancer Society. Atlanta: American Cancer Society, 2009. (book)

Complementary therapies: a guide for people with cancer. Canadian Cancer Society. Toronto: Canadian Cancer Society, 2009. (booklet)

Integrative oncology. Abrams, Donald I; Weil, Andrew T. New York: Oxford University Press, 2009. (book)

Mayo Clinic book of alternative medicine. Mayo Clinic. New York: Time Inc., 2007. (book)

Thinking about complementary and alternative medicine: a guide for people with cancer. National Cancer Institute (U.S.). Baltimore: National Cancer Institute, 2005. (book)

Coping and relaxation

Coming to our senses: healing ourselves and the world through mindfulness. Kabat-Zinn, Jon. New York: Hyperion Audiobooks, 2005. (CD-audiobook)

Dancing in limbo. Halvorson-Boyd, Glenna and Hunter, Lisa. San Francisco: Jossey-Bass, 1995. (book)

Easing into sleep. Miller, Emmett E; Coxon, Robert Haig. Nevada City, CA: Emmett Miller, 2005. (CD)

Guided mindfulness meditation: series 3. Kabat-Zinn, Jon. Lexington, MA: Stress Reduction CDs and Tapes, 2005. (CD)

Heartmindfulness: a guided meditation. Sample, Sarah; Foran, Sydney; Flood, Karen; Nicholson, Kathryn. Vancouver: BC Cancer Agency, Vancouver Centre, 2009. (CD)

Laugh alive!: joyous laughter for listening and participating: pure laughter for fun, health and relaxation. McClelland, Hugh. Vancouver: DreamMaker Studio, 2004. (CD)

Meditations for self-healing and inner power. Borysenko, Joan Z. Carlsbad, CA: Hay House, Inc. 2005. (CD)

Picking up the pieces: moving forward after surviving cancer. Magee, Sherri; Scalzo, Kathy. Vancouver: Raincoast Books, 2006. (book)

Spinning straw into gold. Kaye, Ronnie. New York: Simon and Shuster, 1991. (book)

"Time in" series, 1–7. Smith, Lis. Vancouver: BC Cancer Agency, Patient and Family Counselling, 1987–94. (tapes or CDs)

Intimacy and body image

100 questions and answers about breast cancer sensuality, sexuality, and intimacy. Krychman, Michael L; Spadt, Susan Kellogg; Finestone, Sandra. Sudbury, MA: Jones and Bartlett Publishers, 2011. (book)

Breast cancer husband: how to help your wife (and yourself) through diagnosis, treatment, and beyond. Silver, Marc. Emmaus, PA: Rodale, 2004. (book)

Couples confronting cancer: keeping your relationship strong. Fincannon, Joy L; Bruss, Katherine V; American Cancer Society. Atlanta: American Cancer Society, 2003. (book)

Intimacy after breast cancer: dealing with your body, relationships and sex. Maisano, Gina M. Garden City Park, NY: Square One Publishers, 2010. (book)

Partners in hope: a man's guide to women's breast cancer. Chicago: Bosom Buddies, Inc., 2001. (DVD)

Seventeen short films about breasts. Robertson, Cathryn. Bowen Island, BC: Oystercatcher Film and Television Inc., 2008. (DVD)

Sexuality and cancer: a guide for people with cancer. Canadian Cancer Society. Toronto: Canadian Cancer Society, 2006. (40 page booklet)

Sexuality for the woman with cancer. Rev. ed. Schover, Leslie R. New York: American Cancer Society, Inc., 2010. (booklet online)

Show me: a photo collection of breast cancer survivors' lumpectomies, mastectomies, breast reconstructions and thoughts on body image. 2nd ed. Penn State Milton S. Hershey Medical Center. Hershey, Pa. Milton S. Hershey Medical Center, 2001. (book)

Stand by her: a breast cancer guide for men. Anderson, John W. New York: AMACOM, 2010. (book)

Woman cancer sex. Katz, Anne. Pittsburgh: Oncology Nursing Society Hygeia Media, 2009. (book)

Ties that bind: when your partner has breast cancer. Keeney, Susan Nessim. Los Angeles: Susan Nessim-Keeney/Cancervive, 2006. (DVD)

Personal stories

A safe place: a journal for women with breast cancer. Jennifer Pike. Vancouver: Raincoast Books, 1997. (book)

After the cure: the untold stories of breast cancer survivors. Abel, Emily K; Subramanian, Saskia Karen. New York: New York University Press, 2008. (book)

Breast cancer survivor video series. WomenStories. Madison: Medical Media Associates, Inc. 2006. (DVD)

Cup of comfort for breast cancer survivors: inspiring stories of courage and triumph. Sell, Colleen. Avon, MA: Adams Media, 2008. (book)

How to ride a dragon: women with breast cancer tell their stories. Tocher, Michelle. Toronto: Key Porter Books, 2002. (book)

Life in the balance: my journey with breast cancer. Shapiro, Marla. Toronto: HarperCollins, 2006. (book)

Talking to children

Metu and Lee learn about breast cancer. Sachedina, Shenin. Winter Park, FL: Dr. Shenin Sachedina Medical Educational Products, 2006. (book)

Reaching out to your children when cancer comes to your family: a guide for parents. Slakov, June. Vancouver: BC Cancer Agency.Multi-Media Services, 2007. (book)

When a parent has cancer: a guide to caring for your children. rev. ed. Harpham, Wendy Schlessel. New York: Perennial Curents, 2004. (book)

When cancer joins the family. BC Cancer Agency, Breast Tumour Group; Janes, Karen. Vancouver: BC Cancer Agency, Multi-Media Services, 2007. (DVD)

When your parent has cancer: a guide for teens. National Cancer Institute (U.S.) Baltimore, MD: National Cancer Institute, 2005. (book & book online)

The year my mother was bald. Speltz, Ann; Sternberg, Kate. Washington: Magination Press, 2003. (book)

You are not alone: families touched by cancer. Grayzel, Eva. Easton, PA: Eva Grayzel, 2010. (book)

Lymphedema

100 questions and answers about lymphedema. Thiadens, Saskia R. J. Boston: Jones and Bartlett Publishers, 2010. (book)

Lymphedema and breast cancer: symptom management and exercise after surgery. BC Cancer Agency, Breast Tumour Group; Harris, Susan. Vancouver, BC: BC Cancer Agency. Multi-Media Services, 2006. (DVD)

Lymphedema remedial exercises for the upper extremities. Norton, Steve; Norton School of Lymphatic Therapy. Matawan, NJ: Norton School of Lymphatic Therapy, 2006. (DVD)

Lymphedema: understanding and managing lymphedema after cancer treatment. American Cancer Society. Atlanta: American Cancer Society, 2006. (book)

Advanced breast cancer

100 questions and answers about advanced and metastatic breast cancer. Shockney, Lillie D; Shapiro, Gary R. Boston, MA: Jones and Bartlett Publishers, 2009. (book)

Advanced breast cancer. BC Cancer Agency, Breast Tumour Group; Foran, Sydney; Lohrisch, Caroline. Vancouver: BC Cancer Agency. Multi-Media Services, 2007. (DVD)

Advanced breast cancer: a guide to living with metastatic disease. 2nd ed. Mayer, Musa. Sebastopol, CA: O'Reilly & Associates, Inc., 1998. (book)

More detailed medical information

Clinical guidelines: breast cancer. Clinical practice guidelines for the care and treatment of breast cancer (www.cmaj.ca/cgi/content/full/158/3/DC1). (guideline)

Diseases of the breast. 4th ed. Harris, Jay R. Philadelphia: Lippincott Williams & Wilkins, 2009. (book)

Index

5-FU, 186, 187

A

Acetaminiphen (Tylenol), 189
Activity. *See* Exercise
Addiction concerns,
  in pain management, 271
Adjuvant therapy. *See also*
  Chemotherapy; Hormone therapy;
  Radiation therapy
    overview, 92
    purpose, 129
    recommendations for, 129–130
    start, after surgery, 130
    types
      chemotherapy, 130–131, 180–184
      combined modality, 131
      Herceptin therapy, 131
      hormone therapy, 131
      radiation, 130
Adriamycin (taxorubicin), 186, 195
Advil (ibuprofen), 189
Advocacy, for breast cancer research
  and care
    breaking silence, 299–300, 303
    information dissemination, 300–302
    mutual support, 302–303
    networking, 303–304
Age. *See also* Menopause; Young women,
  and breast cancer
    chemotherapy for breast cancer under
      35, 181, 184
    and risk of breast cancer, 10–11, 13, 14
    and screening mammography, 38–39
Alcohol consumption
    during chemotherapy, 196
    and increased risk of breast cancer

recurrence, 240
link with breast cancer, 13, 17, 21, 237
Allred score, 82, 160
Alternative therapy
  definition, 288
  discussion with conventional doctor,
    294–295
  information, 295
  risks, 294
  types
    biologically based/natural
      products, 290–292
    manipulative and body-based
      practices, 292–293
    mind/body medicine, 292
    whole medical systems, 293
  as unproven by scientific testing, 288,
    289
  use by women with breast cancer,
    288, 289–90
Anastrozole (Arimidex), 14, 22, 163, 169
Androgens, 171–172
Anemia, 188–189
Angiogenesis, 6
Angiosarcoma, 156
Anti-estrogen therapy. *See* Hormone
  therapy
Antiemetics, 190, 191
Appetite. *See* Diet; Nausea
Arimidex (anastrozole), 14, 22, 163, 169
Arm swelling. *See* Lymphedema
Armpit. *See* Axilla (armpit); Axillary
  dissection
Aromasin (exemestane), 14, 22, 163, 169
Aromatase inhibitors
    as adjuvant therapy, 131
    compared with tamoxifen, 163–164

drugs used, 169
not currently recommended as
treatment for DCIS, 135
osteoporosis risk, and use of
supplements, 242–243
for post-menopausal women, 163, 267
for pre-menopausal women, 169
for prevention of cancer recurrence,
14, 135, 163
side effects, 169–170
studies, 22
for treatment for postmenopausal
systemic cancer, 267
ASA (Aspirin), 189
Asian people, breast cancer risk, 18
Aspirin (ASA), 189
Ataxia-telangiectasia, 118
Ativan (lorazepam), 190
Atypia (atypical cells), 8, 15–16, 47
Axilla (armpit). *See also* Axillary
dissection; Lymph nodes
lumps, 49
scarring, as side effect of lymph node
radiation, 155
sensations after surgery, 31
spread of cancer to, 7
Axillary dissection. *See also* Lymph nodes;
Mastectomy
for cancer in axillary lymph nodes,
113, 114–115, 116
"cords," formation of, 215
and lymphedema, 215
for male breast cancer, 287
physical therapy after surgery, 214–215

B

Bellagral, 193
Benadryl (diphenhydramine), 190
Benign growths, 6
Biopsy
core needle, 60–61, 63
definition, 58
fine-needle aspiration, 58–60
fine-wire localization, 66–68
frozen section, 63–64
sentinel node biopsy, 113–114
surgical (open), 61–63
ultrasound-guided needle, 55–56
Birth control. *See* Contraceptives;
Pregnancy
Bisphosphonates, 194, 270, 271
Black cohosh, 193

Black people, and breast cancer, 18
Bleeding
from nipples, 48
as potential side effect of chemotherapy,
189
Bleomycin, 270
Blood clots. *See* Thrombosis
Bones. *See also* Osteoporosis
bone scan, 94, 269
metastases, treatment of, 270
Brachytherapy, 145–146, 148, 152
Brain, treatment of metastases in, 269
Brassiere. *See* Prosthesis, breast
BRCA1 gene. *See also* Family history,
of breast cancer
increased risk of ovarian and breast
cancer, 283
MRI screening for, 49
and risk of developing breast cancer,
284
as strong risk factor in breast and
ovarian cancer, 14, 22
BRCA2 gene. *See also* Family history,
of breast cancer
increased risk of breast cancer in men,
283
increased risk of prostate cancer in
men, 283
MRI screening for, 49
and risk of developing breast cancer,
284
as strong risk factor in breast and
ovarian cancer, 14, 22
Breast. *See also* Breast cancer; Prosthesis,
breast
anatomy, 27–31
changes
with age, 27–28
examination by doctor, 47
symptoms of cancer, 48–49
density, as factor in breast cancer, 15
fat content, 27–28
muscles, 30–31
nerves, 31
physical examination, during staging,
93–94
radiation
discomfort following, 154
during and after pregnancy, 277
red blood vessels (telangiectasia),
154
scarring, 154

Breast cancer. *See also* Biopsy; BRCA1 gene; BRCA2 gene; Ductal carcinoma in situ (DCIS); Invasive breast cancer; Lobular carcinoma in situ (LCIS); Lumps; Metastatic breast cancer; Recurrence, of breast cancer; Risk factors, of breast cancer; Tumours
  appearance
    in mammogram, 51–52
    in ultrasound, 55
  cells
    abnormal division, 8
    characteristics, 74, 80
  classification schemes, 81–84
  development over time, 8
  diagnosis, in pathology report, 75
  estimating risk, 10–11
  incidence, increase in, 10
  lumps, 45, 48
  size, 83
  spread, 6–7, 57, 70
  statistics, 9, 14
  symptoms of, 48–49
  types
    in situ, 8, 76–78
    inflammatory, 84
    invasive, 8, 80–85
    sarcomas, 84–85
  in young women, 279–281
Breast self-examination (BSE)
  advocacy for, 301
  as follow-up to cancer treatment, 259–260
  after partial mastectomy, 119
  screening for breast cancer, 39–40
  techniques, 306–307
Breast specific gamma imaging (BSGI), 42
Breastfeeding, as possible protection against breast cancer, 14
Bruising, as potential side effect of chemotherapy, 189
Buserelin (Suprefact), 162, 170, 195

C

c-erb-B2. *See* HER2 gene over-expression
C-erb-B2 gene. *See* HER2 gene
Calcium deposits, in breast, 52, 76–78
Cancer. *See also* Breast cancer; Coping with cancer; Endometrial cancer; Ovarian cancer; Pathology report; Recurrence, of breast cancer
  cells
    abnormal division, 8
    characteristics, 6–7
    definition, 6
    metastatic, 6
    primary, 6
    secondary, 6
    staging, 93–97
Cancer care system. *See* Health care system
Carboplatin, 187
Carcinoma, definition, 6. *See also* Cancer
Caregivers. *See* Case manager; Family; Friends
Case manager
  advice for, 100–101
  Internet, searching assistance, 100
  questions
    chemotherapy, 178
    surgery, 99
    treatments, 99–100
  role, 98–99
Cells
  atypical cell division, 8
  benign growths, 6
  cancerous, appearance, 74
  malignant growths, 6
  normal division, 5
Cesamet (nabilone), 190
Chemoablation, 269–270
Chemotherapy. *See also* Hair loss; Nausea
  aerobic exercise, during and after treatment, 215–216
  applications
    adjuvant, 92, 130, 175, 176, 177, 180–184
    for high-grade tumours, 279–280
    for locally advanced cancers, 176
    neoadjuvant, 92, 106, 175, 176, 177
    for recurrence of breast cancer, 262, 263
    for symptom relief, 175, 268
    for systemic cancer, 267–268
    for tumours not hormone-sensitive, 183
  basis for therapy recommendation, 181–184
  definition, 175
  drug names and combinations, 186–187
  duration, 177
  fear of, 177–178
  fertility issues, in premenopausal women, 276–277

during pregnancy, 276
purpose, 131
questions regarding treatment, 178
risk and benefit, 178–179, 183–184
side effects, 187–97
Chest. *See also* Breast; Lungs
muscles, 29–30
scarring, as side effect of lymph node
radiation, 156
Children, informing of mother's cancer,
205–206
Classification, of cancer
extent of disease, 83
growth rate, 84
HER2 over-expression, 82
hormone receptors, 81, 82
tumour grade, 82–83
Clinical trials
ethics committees, 298
importance of, 296
steps in testing treatment, 296–297
for systemic cancer, 272
volunteering issues, 272, 298
Clodronate, 194, 270, 271
Clonidine (Dixarit), 166, 193
Colloid infiltrating ductal carcinoma, 81
Comedocarcinoma, 78, 134
Complementary medicine
definition, 288
discussion with conventional doctor,
294–295
information, 295
risks, 294
types
biologically based/natural products,
290–292
manipulative and body-based
practices, 292–293
mind/body medicine, 292
as unproven by scientific testing,
288, 289
use by women with breast cancer,
288, 289–90
Complex physical therapy (CPT) /
complex decongestive therapy (CDP),
for lymphedema, 222–223
Constipation
as side effect of chemotherapy,
190, 191
as side effect of pain management
drugs, 271
Contraceptives. *See also* Pregnancy; Sex

oral
and breast cancer risk, 13, 16, 21
health advantages, 21
not recommended during
chemotherapy, 194
pregnancy prevention, during cancer
treatments, 277
Coping with cancer
emotions, dealing with, 203, 206
end of life decisions, 272
fertility, 209
friends, 208
maintaining hope, 209–210
mental well-being with systemic
cancer, 271
participating in treatment decision-
making, 207–208
Reach to Recovery Program, 207
seeking information, 204–205
sexuality, 209
support groups, 206, 281
telling others, 205–206
Core needle biopsy, 60–61, 63
Cosmetic surgery. *See* Reconstruction,
after breast surgery
Cribiform type, of DCIS, 78
CT-simulator, for radiation therapy, 142–43
Cyclophosphamide (Cytoxan), 186, 187
Cyp2D6 enzyme, 161
Cystosarcoma phylloides, 81, 84–85
Cysts, 47, 53, 54, 59. *See also* Lumps
Cytoxan (cyclophosphamide), 186, 187

D
DCIS. *See* Ductal carcinoma in situ (DCIS)
Decadron (dexamethasone), 190
Denosumab, 270
DepoProvera, 193–194
Dexamethasone (Decadron), 190
Diagnosis of cancer, in pathology report,
75. *See also* Biopsy; Screening, for breast
cancer
Diarrhea
managing with food choices, 242
as side effect of chemotherapy, 190–191
Diet. *See also* Alcohol consumption;
Weight
advice, from registered dietitians, 248
and breast cancer risk, 17, 21
after cancer treatment, 245
during cancer treatment, 240–243
flax seeds, 240

The Healthy Eating Plan for Women,
246–247
link with breast cancer, 237
low-fat, 245
lower fat and calorie, in prevention
of recurrence of cancer, 291
during menopause, 193
plant-based, 238
soybeans and soy supplements, 240
supplements, during treatment, 244
Digital mammography, 47, 52–53
Dimenhydrinate (Gravol), 190
Diphenhydramine (Benadryl), 190
Discharge, nipple, 48
Dixarit (clonidine), 166, 193
Docetaxel (Taxotere), 186, 187
Doctor, family
annual physical examination, 41
follow-up examinations, 257
Doxorubicin, 187
Doxycycline, 270
Drains, after surgery, 123
Drugs. See Aromatase inhibitors;
Chemotherapy; Hormone therapy;
names of drugs
Ductal carcinoma in situ (DCIS)
comedocarcinoma (high-grade DCIS),
78, 134
definition, 76
development, 76–78
recurrence, 148
treatment
partial mastectomy (wide excision)
and radiation, 132–134, 135
partial mastectomy (wide excision)
only, 134
total mastectomy, 133, 135
types, 78, 81
Ducts, milk, 27–28, 29

E

Eat Well, Be Active: What you can do
(Canadian Cancer Society, 2009), 237
Eating Well with Canada's Food Guide,
248
Edema. See Lymphedema
Effexor (venlafaxine), 166, 193
Electric shock sensations, after radiation
therapy, 154
Emend, 190
Emotional effects. See Coping with cancer;
Stress

Endocrine treatment. See Hormone
therapy
Endometrial cancer, 22, 134, 136–137
Environmental risk factors, 16–17, 18
Epirubicin, 186, 187
ER/PR tumour classification
and adjuvant chemotherapy, 181, 182
possible combinations, 160
triple negative cancers, in young
women, 279–280
Estring, 166
Estrogen. See also Hormone therapy;
Tamoxifen
anti-estrogen drugs, 21–22
ER/PR tumour classification, 160
estrogen receptor-positive tumours,
82, 159, 160
lobular carcinomas, as estrogen-
dependent cancers, 81
menopausal symptoms, due to
hormone therapy, 164–168
receptor testing, 63
role in body, 159
triple-negative tumour, adjuvant
chemotherapy for, 181, 182
vaginal creams, concern over use with
hormone therapy, 166
Ethnicity, and risk of breast cancer,
18–19
Etidronate, 194
Evening primrose oil, 193
Evista (raloxifene), 22, 169, 194
Examination, physical
annual, 41
breast, 45–46
breast lump, 47
follow-up, after treatment, 255
follow-up, frequency, 258
Exemestane (Aromasin), 14, 22, 163, 169
Exercise
aerobic, during and after treatment,
215–216
benefits of, 214
during chemotherapy, 196–197
compression sleeve, after axillary
dissection, 221–222
importance, in dealing with
menopause, 193
physical therapy after surgery,
214–215
as possibly lowering risk of breast
cancer, 237

to regain range of shoulder motion,
216–219
regular, as factor in prevention of
breast cancer, 17
strengthening, 220–221

F

Familial breast cancer. *See* BRCA1 gene;
BRCA2 gene; Family history, of breast
cancer
Family history, of breast cancer. *See also*
BRCA1 gene; BRCA2 gene
assessing risks, 14–15
founder mutations, 284
genetic counselling and testing,
284–285
genetic mutations other than BRCA1
and BRCA2, 283
genetic risk assessment criteria, 285
genetic testing for BRCA1 and
BRCA2 genes, 282–283
hereditary cancer surveillance
programs, 285–286
MRI screening, regular, 56
ovarian cancer, risk of, 283
prophylactic mastectomy, 22–23
risk evaluation, 13, 282, 283
risk factors
age at diagnosis, 283, 285
cancer of both breasts, 283–284
family members with breast
cancer, 284, 285
screening, regular, 286
Faslodex (fulvesant), 168–169, 267
Fatigue
during cancer treatment, 241
managing, with food choices, 242
from radiation therapy, 152–153
as side effect of chemotherapy, 196
as symptom of systemic cancer, 268
Femara (letrozole), 14, 163, 164, 169
Fertility, after chemotherapy, 194–195,
281
Fibroadenoma, 53, 54
Fibrocystic disease, 47
Fine-needle aspiration biopsy, 58–60
Fine-wire localization biopsy, 66–68
First Nations people, and breast cancer, 18
Fluid accumulation. *See* Lymphedema
Follow-up, after surgery. *See* Examination,
physical
Food. *See* Diet

Fosamax, 194
Founder mutations, 284
Friends. *See also* Case manager
advice on remedies, 212
emotional support, 211–212
maintaining hope, 209–210
practical support, 210–211
selecting intermediary on your behalf,
211
suggestions of alternative treatments,
290
visitors, during hospitalization, 124
vulnerable times, 212–213
Frozen section biopsy, 63–64
Fulvesant (Faslodex), 168–169, 267

G

G-CSF, 186, 188
Gabapentin (Neurontin), 166, 193
Gas, managing with food choices, 242
General practitioner (GP). *See* Doctor,
family
Genetic testing, for breast cancer, 282–285.
See also BRCA1 gene; BRCA2 gene;
Family history, of breast cancer
Goserelin (Zoladex), 162, 170, 195
Grade, of tumour
adjuvant chemotherapy
recommendations, 181, 182, 183
for predicting tumour growth, 82–83
Granulocyte colony stimulating factor
(G-CSF), 186, 188–189
Gravol (dimenhydrinate), 190

H

Hair loss
as rare side effect of tamoxifen, 168
as side effect of chemotherapy, 187
as side effect of radiation of brain,
152, 269
suggestions for coping, 187
Headache
as rare side effect of tamoxifen, 168
as side effect of fulvesant (Faslodex),
169
as side effect of radiation of brain, 269
Health care system. *See also* Case
manager; Doctor, family; Health care
team; Surgeon
navigation strategies, 98–101
Health care team. *See also* Case manager;
Surgeon

participating in treatment decision-
making, 207–208
selecting leader/navigator for regular
communication, 207
The Healthy Eating Plan for Women,
246–247
Heart
heart disease, contra-indicated for
radiation, 118
side effects of lymph node radiation,
155
Heartburn, as side effect of chemotherapy,
190
HER2 gene. *See also* HER2 gene
over-expression
activity, in pathology report, 74
and invasive breast cancer, 82
testing, tissue removal, 63
triple-negative tumours, adjuvant
chemotherapy for, 181, 182, 183
HER2 gene over-expression
definition, 82
Herceptin as adjuvant therapy,
74, 82, 131
Herceptin for treatment of systemic
cancer, 267
treatment for recurrence of breast
cancer, 262
tumours, adjuvant chemotherapy for,
181–182, 183
her2-neu gene. *See* HER2 gene
Herbal medicine, 291
Herceptin (trastuzumab)
as adjuvant therapy, 74, 131
in combination with chemotherapy,
186–187, 280
in combination with radiation, 268
purpose, 131
specifically targeted to HER2 over-
expressing cancers, 74, 82, 131
for treatment of systemic cancer, 267
Hereditary breast cancer. *See* BRCA1
gene; BRCA2 gene; Family history, of
breast cancer
Herpes, as potential side effect of
chemotherapy, 191
Hidden (occult) cancer, 52
Hormone receptor breast cancers, 82.
See also Estrogen; Hormone therapy;
Progesterone
Hormone replacement therapy (HRT),
and breast cancer risk, 16

Hormone therapy. *See also* Aromatase
inhibitors; Estrogen; HER2 gene over-
expression; Herceptin (trastuzumab);
Hormones; LHRH-agonist drugs; names
of specific drugs; Ovaries; Progesterone;
Tamoxifen
applications
adjuvant, 92, 131, 182
for locally advanced cancer, 176
for recurrence of breast cancer,
262, 263
for systemic cancer, 267
calcium and vitamin D supplements,
242–243
definition, 160
drugs used, 21–22, 131, 161
ER/PR tumour classification, 160
during menopause, 193–194
in post-menopausal women, 162–164
in premenopausal women, 160–62, 280
purpose, 131, 160
side effects, 165–172
types
androgens, 171–172
aromatase inhibitors, 169–170
LHRH agonists, 170–171
progestins, 171
Hormones. *See also* Estrogen; Hormone
therapy; Progesterone
hormone replacement therapy (HRT),
and breast cancer risk, 16
postmenopausal, and risk of breast
cancer, 21
Hospice care, 272
Hospitalization. *See also* Health care team;
Surgery
admission routine, 121
post-surgical issues, 123–124
prosthesis, obtaining, 124–125
recovery from surgery, 121–123
visitors, 124
Hot flushes
relief from, 193–194
as side effect of aromatase inhibitors,
169
as side effect of chemotherapy, 192
as side effect of fulvesant (Faslodex), 169
as side effect of hormone therapy, 22,
162, 165–166
as side effect of tamoxifen, 134, 136,
167
as symptom of menopause, 192

HRT. *See* Hormone replacement therapy (HRT)
Human Epidermal Receptor 2 (HER2) gene. *See* HER2 gene; HER2 gene over-expression
Hyperplasia, 8, 15–16, 47

I

Ibuprofen (Advil), 189
Immune therapies, 292
Implants, after breast surgery. *See also* Reconstruction, after breast surgery
  one-stage silicone filled implant, 229
  tissue expander and implant, 227–228
In situ breast cancer. *See* Ductal carcinoma in situ (DCIS); Lobular carcinoma in situ (LCIS); Paget's disease
Infection
  in arm with lymphedema, 223
  as potential side effect
  of chemotherapy, 188–189
  rare in normal breast, 47
Infiltrating ductal adenocarcinoma, 81
Inflammatory infiltrating ductal carcinoma, 81, 106
Integrative medicine, 288
Intercostal-brachial nerves, 31
Intra-epithelial lobular neoplasia. *See* Lobular carcinoma in situ (LCIS)
Intraductal cancer. *See* Ductal carcinoma in situ (DCIS)
Invasive breast cancer
  appearance, 80
  cell division, 8
  and ductal carcinoma in situ (DCIS), 76, 77, 78
  inflammatory, 84
  and lobular carcinoma in situ (LCIS), 79, 136
  and Paget's disease, 79
  recurrence risks, 256

L

Lapatinib (Tykerb), 82
LCIS. *See* Lobular carcinoma in situ (LCIS)
Letrozole (Femara), 14, 163, 164, 169
Leuprolide (Lupron), 162, 170
LHRH agonists
  in combination with other hormone inhibitors, 170
  purpose, 162, 170
  side effects, 170–171

Ligaments, breast, 28–29
Lipid levels, increase with aromatase inhibitors, 169
Lobular carcinoma in situ (LCIS)
  definition, 78
  recurrence of breast cancer, 14, 148
  treatment, 78–79, 136–137
  types, 81
Lobules, production of breast milk, 27
Locally advanced cancers, 150, 176
Lorazepam (Ativan), 190
Lubricating gels, for vaginal dryness, 166, 191–192
Lumpectomy. *See also* Lumps; Partial mastectomy
  definition, 108
  image-guided excisional biopsy, 62
  MRI follow-up, 56, 143
  radiation follow-up, 92, 141, 145, 147–149
  surgical removal, 110, 276
  treatment, 92
Lumps. *See also* Biopsy; Cysts
  Lumpectomy
  appearance on mammogram, 51, 52
  armpit, 49
  cancerous, 48
  diagnostic ultrasound of, 53–54
  discovery, 45
  examination, 45–46, 47
  fibrocystic disease, 47
  non-cancerous, 45, 47, 52
  size, 52, 83
  solid, 54, 59–60
Lungs
  lung disease, contra-indicated for radiation, 118
  pleural effusion, in recurrent breast cancer, 270
  side effects of lymph node radiation, 155
Lupron (leuprolide), 162, 170
Lupus erythematosus, contra-indicated for radiation, 118
Lymph nodes. *See also* Axilla (armpit); Axillary dissection; Lymphedema; Modified-radical mastectomy; Recurrence, of breast cancer
  cancer spread to, 7, 31, 74, 83
  and chemotherapy, 181, 182, 184
  infection fighting by, 30–31
  location, 30

purpose, 29–30
and radiation therapy, 148–149,
155–156
sentinel node biopsy, 113–114, 116
Lymphatic system
cancer spread, 83
chemotherapy, 184
Lymphedema
after axillary dissection, 215, 222
compression pump, using, 222
compression sleeve, using, 221, 222,
224
preventing, 223–224
after radiation, 155
treating, 222–223
Lymphomas, 81

M
Magnetic resonance imaging (MRI)
diagnostic, 56
and excisional surgical biopsy, 62
for high risk women, as follow-up
after treatment, 258, 259
regular, for women with gene
mutations, 286
screening for breast cancer, 41
Male breast cancer
and BRCA2 gene mutation, 22, 283,
287
increased risk of prostate cancer
with BRCA1 gene, 283
survival rates, 287
symptoms, 287
treatment, 287
Malignant growths, 6. See also Cancer;
Metastases
Mammary carcinoma, 81
Mammograms
abnormal results, 65–66, 68
advocacy for, 301
age, screening recommendations, 38–39
after breast conserving surgery, 259
cancer detection statistics, 10, 40
and core needle biopsy, 61
diagnostic, 50–53
digital, 52–53
and excisional surgical biopsy, 62
"false negative" and "false positive,"
40–41
as follow-up after treatment, 258
after partial mastectomy, 119
procedure, 51

radiation from, 18, 145
recommended frequency, 38–39
screening, 39–40, 40–41, 53
signs of cancer in, 52
usefulness, 35–38
for women with gene mutations, 286
X-ray film, 52
Mammography. See Mammograms
Mammoprint test, 84
Manual lymph drainage (MLD) /
manual lymph treatment (MLT),
for lymphedema, 222
Mastectomy. See also Axillary dissection;
Partial mastectomy; Prosthesis, breast;
Reconstruction, after breast surgery;
Surgery; Total mastectomy
for cystosarcoma phylloides, 84–85
and immediate reconstruction, 112–113
for male breast cancer, 287
partial, 108–110, 132–133
during pregnancy, 276
prophylactic, 22–23, 136, 286
radical, 112
total, 110, 112, 280–281, 286
Maxeran (metoclopramide), 190
Medullary infiltrating ductal carcinoma,
81
Megace (megesterol acetate), 171, 193, 243
Megesterol acetate (Megace), 171, 193, 243
Memory, short-term loss as side effect
of chemotherapy, 196
Men with BRCA2 gene. See Male breast
cancer
Menopause
changes in breast composition, 28
coping strategies, 192–193
definition, 192
early, due to chemotherapy, 192,
276–277
hormone replacement therapy (HRT),
and breast cancer risk, 16
hormone therapy for postmenopausal
systemic cancer, 267
symptoms, as side effect of
chemotherapy, 192–193
symptoms, as side effect of hormone
therapy, 165–174
Menstruation
anti-period drugs, during
chemotherapy, 195
disruption, as side effect of
chemotherapy, 191

early, and risk of breast cancer,
13, 16, 17
Metastases, definition, 6, 80
Metastatic breast cancer. *See* Invasive
breast cancer; Recurrence, of breast
cancer; Systemic cancer
Methotrexate, 186
Metoclopramide (Maxeran), 190
Microarray analysis, 84
Milk ducts
anatomy, 27–28, 29
ductal carcinoma in situ (DCIS), 76–78
Mineral supplements, 244
Mitotic index, 84
Modified-radical mastectomy. *See* Total
mastectomy
Mouth symptoms, as side effect of
chemotherapy, 191, 241
Mucinous infiltrating ductal carcinoma, 81
Mucositis, as side effect of chemotherapy,
191

N

Nabilone (Cesamet), 190
Nausea
managing, with food choices, 241
and nutrition, in systemic cancer, 271
from radiation therapy, 152
as rare side effect of tamoxifen, 168
as side effect of fulvesant (Faslodex),
168
after surgery, 122
treatment, 190
and vomiting, as side effect of
chemotherapy, 190
Necrosis, 6
Neoadjuvant therapy. *See also*
Chemotherapy; Hormone therapy;
Radiation
definition, 92, 106
Neulasta Filgrastim, 188
Neupogen, 188
Neurontin (Gabapentin), 166, 193
Nipples
subcutaneous, skin/nipple-sparing
mastectomy, 110–112
symptoms of breast cancer, 48, 49
Novaldex, 161

O

Occult (hidden) cancer, 52
Oncotype Recurrence Score, 84, 181

Ondansetron (Zofran), 190
Oophorectomy, 162, 286
Osteoporosis
calcium and vitamin D supplements,
166–167, 242–243
risk
with aromatase inhibitors, 169
with chemotherapy, 192–193
hormone therapy, 242–243
with hormone therapy, 166
temporary, with LHRH-agonist drugs,
170–171
treatment, 194
Ovarian cancer
BRCA1 or BRCA2 genes as risk
factors, 14, 22
screening for, as not reliable, 286
Ovarian suppression
effect of LHRH agonist drugs,
170–171
oophorectomy, 162, 286
pituitary suppression, 162
in pre-menopausal women, 162
radiation, 162
Ovaries. *See* Oophorectomy; Ovarian
cancer; Ovarian suppression

P

p27 gene, 84
p53 gene, 84
Paclitaxel (Taxol), 186, 187
Paget's disease
definition, 48, 79
treatment, 79
Pain
management
addiction concerns, 271
from metastases, relief through
radiation, 150
in systemic cancer, 271
as side effect
of aromatase inhibitors, 169
of chemotherapy, 190, 196
of fulvesant (Faslodex), 169
of tamoxifen, 168
stomach, as side effect of
chemotherapy, 190
after surgery, 122–123
as symptom of breast cancer, 48–49
Palliative care, 272
Pamidronate, 270, 271
Papillary type, of DCIS, 78

Partial mastectomy
  for ductal carcinoma in situ (DCIS),
    132–133, 134, 135
  effectiveness in controlling cancer, 116
  follow-up
    lifelong, 133
    radiation, 117, 118–119, 147
    regular medical visits, 119
  personal considerations, 116–117,
    119–120
  surgical issues, 117–118
Pathology report
  features, affecting prognosis and
    treatment, 75
  final diagnosis, 74
  gross description of tissues, 71, 74
  microscopic, 72–73, 74
Patient. *See* Case manager; Coping
  with cancer; Health care team;
  Hospitalization
Pectoralis major muscle, 29–30
Pectoralis minor muscle, 30
Pentagastrin, 188–189
PET. *See* Positron emission tomography
  (PET)
Phlebitis, as side-effect of tamoxifen, 136,
  167. *See also* Thrombosis
Physiotherapy, after surgery, 123, 124.
  See also Exercise
Pituitary gland, suppression in hormone
  therapy, 162. *See also* Hormone therapy;
  LHRH agonists
Plastic surgeon. *See* Reconstruction, after
  breast surgery
Ploidy cells, 84
Positron emission tomography (PET), 57
Pregnancy, and breast cancer
  delay, after hormone treatments, 281
  delivery issues, 276
  diagnosis during pregnancy, 275
  fertility, after chemotherapy, 194–195,
    276–277
  late, as moderate risk factor in breast
    cancer, 14
  normal pregnancy, changes in breast,
    27–28
  pregnancy after treatment, 277–278
  prevention, during chemotherapy,
    194–195
  survival rates, 276
  termination issues, 276
  treatment plan, factors, 275

Preoperative chemotherapy. *See*
  Chemotherapy; Neoadjuvant therapy
Prevention, of breast cancer
  diet, 21
  hormone-suppression drugs, 21–22
  life-style factors, 17, 20–21
  surgical prevention, 22–23
Prochlorperazine (Stemetil), 190
Progesterone. *See also* Hormone therapy
  hormone receptor breast cancers, 82
  progesterone receptor-positive
    tumours, 159, 160
  progestin drugs, 171
  role in body, 159
  triple-negative tumour, adjuvant
    chemotherapy for, 181, 182
Progestins, 171
Prophylactic mastectomy
  as treatment for lobular carcinoma
    in situ (LCIS), 136
  for women with familial breast cancer
    gene, 22–23, 286
Prosthesis, breast. *See also* Reconstruction,
  after breast surgery
  description, 124
  fitted, 125
  medical insurance coverage, 125
  obtaining, 125
  temporary, 124–125
Psychological effects. *See* Coping with
  cancer; Stress

R
Rabeprazole, 190
Race, and risk of breast cancer, 18–19
Radiation
  aerobic exercise, during and after
    treatment, 215–216
  boost, 148
  brachytherapy, 145–146
  in combination with other therapies,
    268
  definition, 141
  dose, 144
  emotional effects, 153
  and increased survival rate after
    mastectomy, 149
  not considered necessary after wide
    excision for very small DCIS, 134
  partial breast radiation, 149–150
  planning session, with CT simulator,
    142, 148

during pregnancy, 276
previous treatment of same breast,
   contra-indicated for, 119
purpose, 141–42
   for breast conservation, in ductal
      carcinoma in situ (DCIS), 132–133
   to decrease pain of bone
      metastases, 270
   following lumpectomy/partial
      mastectomy, 147–149
   following total/modified radical
      mastectomy, 149–150
   for locally advanced cancer,
      150, 176
   for ovarian suppression, 162
   for relief of symptoms from
      metastases, 150–151
   for symptom relief, 268
   for treatment of systemic tumour
      recurrences, 268–269
   use when surgery not advisable, 147
radiated breasts, during and after
   pregnancy, 277
re-treatment options, 146
and recurrence of breast cancer, 262,
   263
risk of cancer, 156
side effects, 149–150, 152–156, 242
strontium use, for bone cancer, 269
timing
   adjuvant therapy, 92, 130
   with breast reconstruction, 234
   after modified radical mastectomy,
      149–150
   after partial mastectomy, 117,
      118–119
treatment
   decision-making, 142
   procedure, 143–145
   session length, 144
when not appropriate, 118–119, 151
when used, 141–142, 147
for young women, 280–281
Radiofrequency ablation, 269–270
Radiotherapy. See Radiation
Raloxifene (Evista), 22, 169, 194
Ranitidine (Zantac), 190
Reach to Recovery Program, 207
Reconstruction, after breast surgery.
   See also Implants, after breast surgery;
   Plastic surgeon; Prosthesis, breast
   delayed, 226, 233–234

factors affecting choice of procedure,
   226
follow-up mammograms, 259
immediate, after mastectomy, 22, 226,
   233, 234, 286
non-interference with breast cancer
   treatment, 225–226
plastic surgeon, referral to, 226
and radiation therapy, 156, 234
timing, 226, 233–234
types
   implant reconstruction, 227–229
   nipple reconstruction, 233
   symmetry surgery, matching other
      breast, 233
   tissue-based reconstruction,
      229–233
Recurrence, of breast cancer. See also
Locally advanced cancers; Metastatic
breast cancer; Systemic cancer
   chemotherapy, risk and benefits,
      178–179, 180–184
   follow-up examinations, 255,
      257–258
   local, 261–262
   after partial mastectomy and radiation,
      262
   patient responsibility for follow-up,
      259–260
   radiation, for relief of symptoms, 147
   risk factors, 256
   symptoms, persistence of, 256–257,
      260
   systemic, 256, 264–272
   treatment considerations, 263
   in young women, 280–281
Relaxation response, 251–252
Remifemin, 193
Research. See Clinical trials
Risk factors, of breast cancer. See also
Family history, of breast cancer;
Prevention, of breast cancer
   age, 10–11, 13, 14
   definition, 12
   estimating, 10–11
   moderate, 13, 15–16
   strong, 13, 14–15
   weak, 13, 16–19

S
S-phase cell number, 84
Sarcomas, 81, 84–85

Scarring
with partial breast radiation, 148–149
after radiation therapy, 154
Scleroderma, contra-indicated for
radiation, 118
Screening, for breast cancer
breast self-examination (BSE), 39–40,
119, 259–260, 306–307
breast specific gamma imaging (BSGI),
42
magnetic resonance imaging (MRI),
41, 56
mammography, 35–39, 40–41
physical examination by medical staff,
41, 45–46
positron emission tomography (PET),
57
recommended frequency, 38–39
thermography, 42
ultrasound, 42, 53–56
Self-examination. See Breast self-
examination (BSE)
Sentinel node biopsy, 113–114, 116, 287
Sex drive
changes during menopause, 194
issues, as side effects of chemotherapy,
191–192
loss with aromatase inhibitors, 169–170
potential effects of cancer diagnosis,
209
Shoulder, exercises to regain range of
motion, 216–219
Side effects. See Aromatase inhibitors;
Chemotherapy; Hormone therapy;
Radiation therapy
Significant other. See Case manager;
Family; Friends
Simple mastectomy. See Total mastectomy
Skin
changes, as side effect of
chemotherapy, 195
effects of radiation therapy, 153–154
symptoms of breast cancer, 47, 48, 49
Smoking, and breast cancer risk, 18
Staging, of cancer. See also Biopsy;
Pathology report
definition, 93
limits of staging system, 94–95
physical examination, 93–94
Stage I, II, III, IV system, 95–96
tests, 94
TNM staging system, 96–97

Stemetil (prochlorperazine), 190
Stress. See also Coping, with cancer
assessing symptoms, 249–250
at cancer diagnosis, 249
definition, 20
reducing, 20–21, 250–252
relief, during menopause, 193
Strontium, 269
Support groups
for coping with cancer, 206
for young women, with breast cancer,
281
Suprefact (buserelin), 162, 170, 195
Surgeon
breast, 106, 121, 122
plastic surgeon, 225–226, 234
Surgery. See also Adjuvant therapy;
Biopsy; Hospitalization; Mastectomy;
Neoadjuvant therapy; Oophorectomy;
Reconstruction, after breast surgery
aim, 116
decisions
choosing a surgeon, 106
choosing partial or total
mastectomy, 116–120
considering options, 107–108
informing yourself, 105
lymph nodes, removal during breast
surgery and assessment, 113–115
and neoadjuvant chemotherapy, 106
post-surgery issues
drains, 114–115, 123
emotional issues, 124
follow-up treatment (adjuvant
therapy), 129–31
healing, 123–124
hematoma, 124
infection, 124
information, for going home, 123
nausea, 122
notifying significant other, 122
numbness, 124
pain, 122–123
physiotherapy, 123, 124
recovery, 121–123
purpose
for breast cancer during
pregnancy, 276
for locally advanced cancer, 176
for phylloides tumour, 280
for systemic recurrence of cancer,
269–270

sutures, 123
types
    breast conservation, 108–110
    breast removal, 110–112
    when appropriate, 105–106
Surgical (open) biopsy
    excisional (complete removal of lump),
        61–62
    incisional (partial removal of lump),
        62–63
    by surgeon experienced in breast
        cancer surgery, 63
Survival rates. See Staging, of cancer
Sutures, after surgery, 123
Swallowing difficulty, managing with
    food choices, 242
Swelling. See also Lymphedema
Systemic cancer. See also Metastatic breast
cancer
    common sites, 265
    factors, 264–265
    metastases, definition, 6, 80
    palliative care, 272
    self-care
        mental well-being, 271
        nutrition, 271
        and pain management, 271
    survival rates, 266, 272
    symptoms, 265
    treatment
        for bone metastases, 270
        chemotherapy, 176–177, 267–268
        clinical trials, 272
        factors, 266–267
        for fluid accumulation, 270
        goals, 265–266
        hormone therapy, 267
        options, 106
        radiation, 150–151, 268–259

T
Tamofen (tamoxifen). See Tamoxifen
Tamoxifen
    applications
        as adjuvant therapy, 131, 161, 163
        male breast cancer, 287
        prevention of breast cancer,
            21, 286
        reduction of breast cancer
            recurrence, 14, 134
        treatment of estrogen-receptor
            positive DCIS, 134

treatment of postmenopausal
    systemic cancer, 267
benefits, for post-menopausal women,
    163
pregnancy, avoidance during treatment,
    168
side effects, 21–22, 134–135, 136,
    167–168
studies, on optimal treatment period,
    164
Taste, affected by chemotherapy, 241
Taxol (paclitaxel), 186
Taxorubicin (Adriamycin), 186
Taxotere (Doxetaxel), 186, 187
Telangiectasia, 154
Tests. See Biopsy; Magnetic resonance
    imaging (MRI); Mammograms;
    Positron emission tomography (PET);
    Ultrasound
Thermography screening, for breast cancer,
    42
Throat
    managing sore throat with food
        choices, 242
    side effects of lymph node radiation,
        155
Thrombosis
    as side effect of anti-estrogen drugs,
        22, 134
    as side effect of tamoxifen, 20–21, 136,
        167
Tiredness. See Fatigue
Tissue-based reconstruction, after breast
surgery
    myocutaneous flap, involving
        latissimus dorsi muscle, 229–230
    transverse rectus abdominus muscle
        (TRAM) flap, 230–232
Total mastectomy. See also Reconstruction,
    after breast surgery
    definition, 110
    effectiveness in controlling cancer,
        116
    for extensive ductal carcinoma in situ
        (DCIS), 133
    personal considerations, 117
    procedure, 112
    surgical issues, 117–119
TRAM (transverse rectus abdominus
    muscle) flap, 230–233
Trastuzumab (Herceptin). See Herceptin
    (trastuzumab)

Treatment, of breast cancer. *See also*
  Chemotherapy; Hormone therapy;
  Radiation therapy; Surgery
    adjuvant therapies, 92
    decisions, 91
    neoadjuvant chemotherapy, 92
    surgery, 92
Trelstar (triptorelin), 162, 170
Triglyceride levels, increase with
  aromatase inhibitors, 169
Triptorelin (Trelstar), 162, 170
Tubular infiltrating ductal carcinoma, 81
Tumours. *See also* Biopsy; Cancer; Cells;
  Pathology report
    ER/PR classification, 160
    large, chemotherapy for, 184
Tykerb (lapatinib), 82
Tylenol (acetaminiphen), 189

U
Ultrasound
    and core needle biopsy, 61
    diagnostic, 53–56
    and excisional surgical biopsy, 62
    as follow-up to mammogram, 259
    regular, for women with gene
      mutations, 286
    ultrasound-guided needle biopsy,
      55–56

V
Vagi-Fems, 166
Vaginal dryness
    as side effect of aromatase inhibitors,
      169
    as side effect of chemotherapy,
      191–192, 193
    as side effect of hormone therapy,
      166
Vascular system, extent of cancer spread,
  83
Venlafaxine (Effexor), 166, 193
Visitors. *See* Friends
Vitamins
    calcium and vitamin D supplements
      for osteoporosis prevention,
      242–243
    caution against antioxidants during
      cancer treatment, 290–291
    supplements, during treatment, 244
    vitamin D for cancer prevention, 243
Vomiting. *See* Nausea

W
Weight. *See also* Diet; Nutrition
    and development of lymphedema after
      axillary dissection, 223
    as factor in breast cancer, 13, 17, 237
    gain
        during breast cancer treatment,
          243
        as side effect or hormone therapy,
          167
    healthy
        calculating BMI, 238–239
        as factor in preventing recurrence
          of cancer, 291
        importance of, 238
    managing
        after treatment, 245
        during treatment, 244
Wide excision mastectomy. *See* Partial
  mastectomy

X
X-rays, and breast cancer risk, 18

Y
Young women, and breast cancer.
  See also Family history, of breast cancer
    HER2 gene over-expressive cancers,
      279, 280
    high-grade and aggressive tumours,
      279, 280
    occurrence, 279
    phylloides tumours, 280
    pregnancy delay, after hormone
      treatments, 281
    recommendations for adjuvant
      therapies, 181, 184
    support groups, 281
    survival rates, 280
    treatment, 279–280
    "triple negative" cancers, 279, 280

Z
Zantac (ranitidine), 190
Zofran (ondansetron), 190
Zoladex (goserelin), 162, 170, 195
Zolendronic acid, 270